unSHAKEable

A Proven Plan To
Crush Anxiety,
Defeat Overwhelm,
And Conquer The Fears
That Freak You Out

UNSHAKEABLE

A Proven Plan To
Crush Anxiety,
Defeat Overwhelm,
And Conquer The Fears
That Freak You Out

JASON & TORI
BENHAM

Bestselling Authors of *Beauty In Battle*

Unshakeable: *A Proven Plan To Crush Anxiety, Defeat Overwhelm, And Conquer The Fears That Freak You Out*

© 2025 by Jason and Tori Benham

Learn more about Tori and Jason at JasonAndTori.com.

Published in Charlotte, North Carolina, by Benham Media.

Unless otherwise indicated, Scripture quotations are taken from the Holy Bible, New International Version, and New American Standard Bible.

New International Version, NIV. © 1973, 1978, 1984, 2011 by Biblica, Inc. Used by permission of Zondervan. All rights reserved worldwide.

New American Standard Bible, NASB. © 1960, 1962, 1963, 1968, 1971, 1972, 1973, 1975, 1977, 1995 by The Lockman Foundation. Used by permission.

Interior & cover design by Shabbir Badshah

ISBN: 979-8-9923386-2-1
Audio Book ISBN: 979-8-9923386-4-5
E-Book ISBN: 979-8-9923386-3-8

Printed in the United States of America

Bulk purchases available. Contact through JasonAndTori.com.

DEDICATION

This book is dedicated to you—the one searching for peace in the middle of the storm. Maybe you're the one battling anxiety, or maybe someone you love is. Either way, you're the reason we wrote Unshakeable. *Every story, every step, and every truth in these pages was written with you in mind. We've been there, and we want you to know there is hope.*

You don't have to stay stuck. Freedom is possible—and it starts right here.

MORE BOOKS BY **THE BENHAMS**

BEAUTY IN BATTLE
Winning In Marriage By Waging A War

MARRIAGE A TO Z
30 Days To Relational Transformation

BOOKS BY JASON AND HIS BROTHER, DAVID:

WHATEVER THE COST
Facing Your Fear, Dying To Your Dreams, And Living Powerfully

LIVING AMONG LIONS
How To Thrive Like Daniel In Today's Babylon

MIRACLE IN SHREVEPORT
*A Memoir Of Baseball, Fatherhood,
And The Stadium That Launched A Dream*

BOLD AND BROKEN
Becoming The Bridge Between Heaven And Earth

EXPERT OWNERSHIP
Launching Faith-Filled Entrepreneurs Into Greater Freedom And Success

EXPERT OWNERSHIP LISTENING PRAYER JOURNAL
Get The Master's Mind On Your Life And Business

BRACE FOR IMPACT
A Biblical Blueprint For Building Wealth And Breaking Strongholds

Visit BenhamBrothers.com/Books for more information.

TABLE OF CONTENTS

66

*"Therefore let us be grateful for receiving a kingdom that **cannot be shaken**, and thus let us offer to God acceptable worship, with reverence and awe, for our God is a consuming fire."*

(Hebrews 12:28-29)

"When God spoke at Sinai, God's voice shook the earth. When your world is shaking, it's because God is talking. We tend to focus our attention on our circumstances. But God wants your attention on him. He has something he wants to tell you, something he wants you to learn.

What's the goal of the shaking? The removal of what can be shaken ... so that what is not shaken might remain. When things are shaking, God is trying to eliminate a hindrance in your life. He's attempting to loosen your grip on created physical things so that you'll grasp tightly onto eternal things instead. The shaking process isn't fun—especially when you don't want to let go. But, remember: God is treating you like his child and not his enemy."

–Dr. Tony Evans[1]

FOREWORD

If you sit down with Jason and Tori Benham, it won't take long to see why people are drawn to them. They love God deeply and care for people genuinely, and it shows in every interaction. Jason, a former pro baseball player, brings the intensity of an athlete. Tori, a faithful wife and fierce truth-teller, brings the strength of a woman who's walked through the fire and come out stronger. They're bold. Passionate. A little wild. And fully surrendered to Jesus.

But here's what might surprise you. For all their strength, success, and Scripture-filled confidence, they were blindsided by something they never saw coming: anxiety. It hit Jason like a freight train before a speaking engagement—his heart racing, hands shaking, panic overwhelming his entire body. Meanwhile, Tori had her own long battle with fear. Her struggles were more private and unseen, but always present. What they experienced wasn't just emotional. It was physical. It was spiritual. And without warning, it was debilitating.

But rather than hiding it, pretending, or powering through it, Jason and Tori turned to God. They went to His Word. They fought through the fear. They renewed their minds with truth. They did the hard, holy work of healing—together.

That's what makes this book special. *Unshakeable* isn't theory, it's their testimony. Their fight. Their faith in the fire. To be clear, it's not a clinical breakdown of anxiety. It's a call to spiritual war, and a reminder that you don't have to fight alone. It's raw, real, Christ-centered, and deeply practical.

What I love most is how Jason and Tori write with honesty from the middle of the battle, not the end. They don't pretend to have it all figured out. But they do know the God who brings peace in the storm. And in these pages, they hand you the same tools that helped them push back the darkness and reclaim the life God meant for them to live.

I sincerely love Jason and Tori—not just for their passion, but for their faithfulness. They are two of the most loving people I know. Their faith is so real, it's contagious. The way they love God overflows into the way they love people, and their lives have inspired me to lead with more courage and love. I've learned so much from them, and I believe you will too.

If you're overwhelmed, exhausted, anxious, or afraid, and your alarm keeps going off for reasons you can't explain—this book is for you. And if you love someone who's struggling but don't know how to help, it's for you too.

Because freedom isn't just possible—it's promised. And your journey begins right here.

Craig Groeschel
Senior Pastor of Life.Church
Author of *Winning the War in Your Mind*

INTRODUCTION

SOUND THE ALARM

"I am an old man and have known a great many troubles,
but most of them never happened."
–Mark Twain

When our kids were little, our master bedroom was upstairs, right alongside theirs. Tori loved knowing we were just a few steps away—it made her feel safe having everyone on the same floor. We had an alarm system downstairs, which gave us extra peace of mind. If an uninvited guest (aka intruder) showed up, we'd be alerted before they got too comfortable.

One night, around 2 AM, we were startled awake by the sound of glass shattering—it sounded as if someone had just smashed a window—followed by our alarm blaring louder than a fire truck in the living room. Instantly, we jolted upright and leaped out of bed like we'd just found a mouse under the covers.

I vividly remember the feeling in my body—a surge of energy hit me, almost electric, my heart slammed against my chest, and my breathing instantly turned shallow and rapid. My muscles tensed, coiled and ready to spring into action and fight off whatever danger my brain had decided was about to burst through the door. Heat rushed to my face, and my stomach felt like it had dropped ten stories in an elevator.

In a split second, my body had launched into full-blown fight-or-flight mode. I was convinced I was about to defend my home like an action hero despite having no plan beyond looking intimidating and hoping for the best.

I had no idea what to do, so I did the first thing that came to mind—I yelled at the top of my lungs, "HEY! Get out of here!!!!" and, for reasons unknown, followed it up with a deep, guttural roar that sounded like an ancient dragon straight out of a sci-fi movie. (Tori: *He really did growl.*) Apparently, when survival mode kicks in, dignity goes out the window.

Then, I army-crawled down the hallway toward my kids' rooms while Tori called 911. Shockingly, everyone was still sound asleep, completely unfazed by the chaos. That didn't last long because I frantically woke them up and told them to run to our room. They bolted down the hall at full speed, just as freaked out as we were, while the alarm blared.

Once we got all the kids into the room, I heard Tori on the phone with the 911 operator. Her voice shook, and her face was as white as a pillowcase as she gripped the phone. I slammed the door shut, locked it, and threw my weight against it as if I was the only thing standing between my family and certain doom. The operator told us to go into the bathroom and lock the door while she sent the police.

Meanwhile, the alarm was still blaring, each pulse screaming that someone was in our house, lurking in the shadows, waiting to dismember us one by one. My brain was fully spiraling, the kids were losing it, and Tori—well, let's just say it took her over a year to recover from this night.

The police got there fast, thankfully. They pulled around to the back of the house, which worked in our favor since our bathroom window faced that direction. As soon as they stepped out, flashlights in hand, they started scanning the house. I opened the window and yelled, letting them know we were huddled in the bathroom. They told us to stay put while they made their way around the house, shining their lights into every room, checking for whatever—or whomever—had set off the chaos.

They came back around and let us know there was no sign of forced entry, which meant it was *probably* safe for me—*not* Tori, *not* my oldest son—to head downstairs and turn off the alarm. So, like the brave warrior I never trained to be, I crept out of the bathroom, cracked open the bedroom door, and made my way down the stairs, still fully prepared for hand-to-hand combat if it came to that.

As soon as I flipped on the light, I spotted the culprit: a motion detector affixed to the kitchen wall was now shattered on the floor. After unlocking the door and letting the police inside, I bent down to inspect the wreckage. Turns out, the adhesive on the back had given up on life, causing the detector to fall and break (aka, the "glass-shattering" sound that had sent my entire nervous system into meltdown mode).

I gotta be honest—I was *embarrassed.* Here I was, a grown man, standing in my kitchen with two other grown men (who face real danger for a living), all of us chuckling over what a massive debacle this had been. We stepped outside, still laughing, only to see Tori leaning out the upstairs window, frantically yelling, "Are we safe?!"

We let her know that all was OK and that she and the kids could come downstairs. Not long after, all the kids huddled in our bed and we drifted off to sleep together as a family.

It was a night we'll never forget. We still laugh (and cringe) about it to this day, and now, as you can see, we're writing about it. Why? Because it's the perfect example of how our bodies react the same way. Just like our house had an alarm system designed to alert us to danger—real or imagined—our bodies come equipped with their own built-in security system.

God wired us with an internal alarm system to help keep us safe. When a potential threat arises, our bodies respond instinctively—heart pounding, muscles tightening, senses sharpening—all designed to prepare us for action. This built-in response enables us to react quickly in dangerous situations. But just like my *kitchen motion detector meltdown,* sometimes the alarm goes off when there's no real danger.

Fear triggers the alarm; it's the signal that sets everything into motion, whether there's an actual threat or not. It doesn't need solid evidence or a logical reason—just the *possibility* of something going wrong is enough to sound the alarm. And once fear pulls that trigger, your body doesn't stop to fact-check; it just reacts.

This system is a gift from God. If we didn't have it, we'd be like the toddler who wants to put a fork into an electrical outlet. Our internal alarm system is designed to protect us, helping us recognize and develop a healthy sense of fear of real dangers. On a hike in the woods and almost step on a copperhead snake? Healthy fear—sound the alarm! In a busy airport with your two-year-old, and she wanders off for a few seconds? Healthy fear—sound the alarm!

Can you imagine what it would be like if we didn't experience fear in those moments? We'd step on the snake. We'd let our innocent kid roam the airport. But God didn't wire us that way. He designed our alarm system to alert us to real danger—so we'd feel fear, act on it, and move toward safety. Fear itself isn't the problem; it's a survival tool.

Imagine if someone had actually broken into our house that night. The alarm system would have done what it was designed to do—alert us to real danger and put Tori and me in a position to protect ourselves and our family.

Fear isn't the enemy. *Anxiety-induced* fear is. This fear isn't based on real threats but on imagined ones created in the mind. When anxiety takes over, it hijacks our fear response, constantly triggering the alarm for danger that doesn't truly exist.

Here's the problem: our bodies don't know the difference between real and imagined threats, so we react the same way to both. That's how anxiety keeps us trapped—responding to worst-case scenarios that only exist in our heads.

It's like a smoke detector that goes off when you burn toast. There's no fire, no real danger—just a little extra crisp on your breakfast. But your alarm doesn't know the difference, so it treats the situation like a five-alarm blaze. That's exactly what anxiety does in our minds. It whispers, *"What if?"* and suddenly, our bodies prepare for catastrophe, even when nothing is truly wrong.

The real issue isn't the alarm itself; it's what keeps setting it off. When anxiety hijacks our fear response and keeps pulling the alarm for false threats, we start living in a constant state of stress, treating everyday situations like life-or-death emergencies. Over time, our bodies forget how to turn the alarm off, trapping us in an exhausting cycle of anxiety.

Just like Tori, locked in the bathroom, yelling down to the police, "Are we safe?" Anxiety traps us in the same cycle of uncertainty. It keeps us stuck, constantly questioning, "Is everything okay? Am I safe?" And until we can answer that with a firm, "Yes, God is in control," we remain just as locked up in fear as Tori and the kids were in that bathroom.

But I'm getting ahead of myself.

The real question is, what pulled the trigger on the alarm—was it a real threat, or was anxiety feeding you a lie? Was it reality, or was it anxiety?

The problem isn't the alarm.
The problem isn't fear.
The problem is what triggered the fear in the first place.

And that's what we're about to uncover in this book.

WAKE UP CALL

I know the feeling of being trapped by anxiety all too well. It happened to me three years ago, just before I stepped on stage with my twin brother to speak at a pro-life event in Vidalia, GA—home of the sweetest onion you'll ever taste and, ironically, the place where I nearly crumbled under the weight of anxiety for the first time.

We were kicking back at our table, talking with the people around us, and doing our best to choke down some not-so-tender filets when my heart started racing out of nowhere. My face got hot, and before I knew it, my fork was on the table, and I was leaning back in my chair, trying to figure out why I suddenly felt like I was melting. Beads of sweat popped up on my forehead, a wave of heat wrapped around me, and everything in the room started closing in like I was looking through a tunnel.

I grabbed my glass of ice water from the table and started gulping it down, then pressed the cold glass against my forehead, hoping it would snap me out of whatever was happening. We were supposed to take the stage in five minutes, but at that moment, public speaking was the last thing on my mind. I wanted out. I didn't care who expected to hear us talk or how many people would be disappointed—I just wanted to disappear.

I thought about getting up and heading to the bathroom, but I was genuinely afraid to stand up. Every instinct told me I was about to pass out. (Side note: I still hold the honor of being the only guy out of 180 players in the Baltimore Orioles organization to pass out while giving blood during the 1998 Spring Training physicals. Safe to say, I've never lived that one down.)

My mind was racing—*What if I pass out on stage? Will someone capture it on video? Will it go viral? Will I forever be known as a meme?* I had no idea how I was supposed to stand up and speak in front of a packed room when I could barely sit upright at my table without feeling like I was going to hit the floor.

At that moment, I had no clue what was happening, no idea what was coming next, and zero confidence in how I would get through it. But there was one thing I did know—I was God's kid, and He was there to help me. So I whispered a prayer, asking for His strength, and then clung to Philippians 4:6-7:

"Do not be anxious about anything, but in everything by prayer and supplication with thanksgiving let your requests be made known to God. And the peace of God, which surpasses all understanding, will guard your hearts and your minds in Christ Jesus."

I started breathing slowly and deeply, reminding myself that if God had called me to this, He would give me the strength to do it. At the same time, I went to work on a piece of chocolate cheesecake because somewhere in the fog of my panic, I remembered that people can pass out if they're low on sugar. (Tori: *That's a convenient excuse to eat dessert, in my opinion.*)

I started feeling a little better, but I still wasn't myself. The burn in my chest and the pit in my stomach felt like nothing I'd ever experienced before. As David and I walked toward the stage, I grabbed another cold glass of ice water and brought it up there, hoping it would keep me from melting down in front of the audience.

I stood next to my brother, knees shaking, gripping the podium like a walker keeping me upright. I managed to get through my part of the talk, but when David started speaking, and I stood there listening, I again felt like I was about to hit the floor. Every few minutes, I'd take a sip of my ice water, then press the chilled glass against my forehead, hoping it would keep me from completely unraveling.

To this day, I wonder what the audience was thinking. It was probably something like, *"Why does this guy look so pale? And why is he holding that water glass like it's his emotional support animal?"*

By the grace of God, I made it through. As the night went on, those insane feelings and sensations slowly faded. But just when I thought I was in the clear, the minute we got into the car to head home, they all came rushing back.

It was so bad that I turned to David and said, "You're driving." I was genuinely afraid that if I stayed behind the wheel, I'd pass out, and we'd both die.

I was completely confused. What was happening to me? I was a professional speaker—I could do that in my sleep. And I had been driving for three decades without a problem. Now, suddenly, I couldn't do either one without feeling like I was about to keel over and die?!

That night was a wake-up call I couldn't ignore. At the time, I didn't fully understand what had happened, but looking back, it was clear—I had a full-blown anxiety attack. Some people call it a panic attack. Whatever label you slap on it, it was miserable.

The scariest part? The very thing I was good at, the thing I was called to do, suddenly felt impossible. And I had no idea how to fix it.

Over the next few weeks and months, the attacks kept coming. They would hit at the most random times—while driving, while sitting at home, even in moments when I should have been completely relaxed. My internal alarm system was stuck on full-blown, five-alarm-fire mode—blaring nonstop—and I didn't know how to turn it off.

Thankfully, Tori saw what I couldn't see. She stepped in and rescued me in a way I didn't even know I needed. She didn't just help me through it—she nursed me back to health. She studied, prayed, researched, and walked beside me as I fought to understand what was happening and, more importantly, how to break free from it.

That's why we wrote this book together. While it's written in my voice, Tori taught me the lessons. She helped me understand anxiety, how it works, and how to fight back. What we learned together completely changed my life.

Now, we're sharing it with you—so you can break free, too. We wrote it to get you out of that locked room or whatever prison anxiety has trapped you in, convincing you that danger is ahead and you're not safe.

In these pages, we will dig deep into what's triggering the alarm in your mind—what's setting off panic over things that may not even be a real threat. Because here's the truth: anxiety is a liar, and Satan is the one pulling its strings. He convinces you that you're powerless, that disaster is around the corner, and that peace is some mystical thing reserved for people who drink herbal tea and do yoga at sunrise.

None of that is true. You can crush anxiety, defeat overwhelm, and conquer the fears that freak you out. And we're here to help you do it.

I should probably clarify something—we're not "anxiety experts" with a bunch of fancy degrees hanging on our walls. We're just regular people who got hit with anxiety out of nowhere, suffered through it, and, by the grace of God, figured out how to break free.

We've been where you are. This is personal for us.

Tori battled fear for years—quiet, constant, and always lurking beneath the surface. One fear kept her paralyzed until she finally chose to face it head-on. She didn't fight with willpower; she fought with truth. And over time, that fear began to lose its grip. She'll tell you the story later on.

So, we know how frustrating it is to feel trapped in a cycle of fear with no idea how to get out.

But we didn't stay stuck. And you don't have to either.

If God brought us through it, He can do the same for you.

What we're about to share with you isn't theory. It's a proven, practical method that helped us get out of anxiety's grip and stay free.

To help you get there, we'll take you to a dusty baseball field, where a pitcher's fastball taught me one of the greatest lessons of my life. You'll tag along on a fancy resort trip, where the highlight wasn't the elegant dinner party—it was the public restroom. We'll hop into a runaway car, where the gas pedal was pinned, and the brakes were useless. And you'll sit next to me on a plane ride, where I discovered that the pit in my stomach wasn't anxiety at all, but something much, much worse.

We've broken this book into two parts to make it as practical and straightforward as possible.

Part One dives into four key areas of anxiety—what it is, how it works, what it does to you, and what causes it. Most books on anxiety are way too technical, and the last thing you need when you're struggling is a bunch of complicated explanations. So, we've worked hard to break it down in a way that's easy to understand and apply.

Once we've laid a solid foundation and exposed anxiety for the fraud it is, we'll move on to Part Two, where you'll learn the powerful three-step plan we developed to break anxiety's grip and plant yourself firmly in a place of peace and confidence.

So, if you're tired of fear running your life, if you're ready to fight back against the enemy's lies, and if you want to experience real, lasting peace—keep reading. The key to your breakthrough is in the pages ahead.

Freedom isn't just possible—it's yours for the taking.

BEFORE YOU BEGIN

Hey there—real quick before you jump in…

This isn't the kind of book you binge in one weekend like a Netflix series. (Well, you *could*, but you'll probably finish it feeling like you just hit up an all-you-can-eat Chinese buffet and went six plates too deep. We've been there. It's not pretty.)

Instead, think of *Unshakeable* like a workout for your soul. You wouldn't try to do 100 squats, run 10 miles, and deadlift a Prius all in one day unless you enjoy pulling hamstrings.

So here's the play:

Take your time.

Read a chapter, let it marinate, and give it time to settle in.

Even better, talk it out with someone if you can.

We wrote it to be slowly digested, not devoured.

Trust us, you can't crush anxiety by flipping pages fast. But if you walk through this book with intention and pace yourself, you'll come out stronger, steadier, and ready for anything.

Now take a deep breath…

Here we go.

PART ONE

THE PROBLEM

"To defeat an enemy, you must know them."
–Grand Admiral Thrawn, Star Wars

If you don't understand what anxiety is, how it operates, and how it affects you, then it will always have the upper hand. But when you take the time to study it—to recognize its patterns and uncover its origin—you position yourself to fight back effectively.

Sun Tzu's timeless classic, *The Art of War*, has been studied by generals and military strategists for centuries. It emphasizes that warriors must first understand their enemy before entering the battlefield. The fight against anxiety is no different.

If you don't recognize anxiety for what it truly is, you'll waste energy fighting the wrong battles. You'll try to fix external circumstances when the real war is happening in your mind and heart.

In Part One, we will focus on four key questions about anxiety:

- What is it?
- How does it work?
- What are its effects?
- What are its root causes?

Anxiety is a word we hear all the time, but what is it actually? We'll break it down in simple terms—no complicated medical jargon—just a clear, practical understanding of what anxiety is at its core. Because let's be real, if we needed a PhD to understand it, we'd all just stay anxious trying to figure it out.

Once we understand what anxiety is, the next step is figuring out how it works. Why does a single thought spiral into full-blown panic? How does your nervous system work, and why do hormones like adrenaline and cortisol take over, convincing your body that disaster is imminent?

Of course, anxiety doesn't just stay in your head; it affects every part of your life. So we'll examine what anxiety does to you—how it hijacks your brain, distorts your emotions, and perverts pressure to steal your peace, limit your potential, and keep you from fully living the life God intended for you.

Then, we'll explore the root causes of anxiety and identify its source using a simple, four-part acronym—**STOP**—that breaks it down into key areas to examine. This section will help you identify the underlying factors behind anxiety and pinpoint what might be fueling yours.

By the time Part One is done, you'll have a solid understanding of what anxiety is, how it works, what it does, and where it comes from—laying the foundation for Part Two: learning how to overcome it for good.

To set the stage, let me take you to a Little League baseball field where the sun was shining, the crowd was cheering, and every kid was eager to play—except for one.

CHAPTER 1

YOU'RE INVITED

*"Anxiety is a thin stream of fear trickling
through the mind. If encouraged,
it cuts a channel into which all other
thoughts are drained."*
—Arthur Somers Roche

———

When I was a kid, baseball was my world. My brother and I quickly
built a reputation as two of the best players in our city. (Tori:
Nothing wrong with a little humble brag.) But no amount of talent or
trophies could help me overcome my greatest fear: facing Brent Murphy.

Brent was *that* guy—the pitcher every kid dreaded. To a young kid, it
felt like he was throwing 500 mph! Just seeing him warm up on the
mound was enough to make your knees buckle. I wasn't the only one.
Half our team would rather face a swarm of bees than step into the
batter's box against Brent. Even spotting his team on the schedule made
you want to pull the covers over your head and call in sick for the season.

Every time I thought about facing him, I could almost feel the sting of a
baseball smashing into my head. I pictured myself collapsing dramatically
to the ground and hearing the sirens of an ambulance racing to the field.
In vivid detail, I imagined being hoisted onto a stretcher, rushed to the
hospital, and, yes, my poor parents grieving at my funeral.

It was bad.

Now, here's the thing—Brent was a solid pitcher. To my knowledge, he hadn't hit a single batter all season. But logic didn't matter to my anxious little mind. My fear took the wheel, hit the gas, and drove straight into a nightmare that felt as real as if it had already happened.

Anxiety doesn't need facts; it just needs an imagination.

The day of the game finally arrived, and I found myself more excited about the thought of it being over than actually playing. I wasn't focused on the game—I just wanted to survive. But I bravely put on my uniform, hopped into my parents' car with my brother, and off we went to the ballpark.

I saw the other team warming up when we got to the field. The sight of Brent sent a chill down my spine. I had secretly hoped he'd come down with the flu or had to miss the game for some miraculous reason. No such luck.

The game started, and I was batting third. The first hitter struck out—no surprise there. As I stood in the on-deck circle, waiting for my turn, my legs felt shaky and unsteady. My heart was racing, and I started feeling lightheaded. At the time, I had no idea these were the classic signs of anxiety.

Every time Brent fired a pitch, I could hear the sharp whiz of the ball slicing through the air and the loud pop of it hitting the catcher's mitt. With each sound, my worst fears felt closer to becoming reality.

So I did what any reasonable kid would do at that moment—I faked being sick. I walked over to my coach, clutching my stomach, and told him I wasn't feeling well and thought I might throw up.

Without hesitation, he took me out of the game and told me to sit with my mom. I placed my helmet and bat back in the dugout and made the slow walk toward her. As I passed by, I glanced at my dad. The look on his face said it all—he always taught us kids to face our fears, but on this day, I had let fear win, and we both knew it.

Sitting there next to my mom, watching my teammates face what I was too afraid to, a wave of guilt hit me. Deep down, I knew what I had done. But in that moment, the fear felt too big to fight. There was just no way I could stand in that batter's box and willingly put myself in the line of fire.

At that moment, I felt completely powerless. It didn't matter that I was one of the best players on the team. My skills, my past successes—none of it made a difference. When I started projecting fear into my future, I turned from a player into a spectator. I spent the rest of the game sitting in the stands, weighed down with regret for giving in to fear and abandoning my teammates.

The result? I was no longer part of the action. I couldn't change the outcome and had no influence. I had become nothing more than a powerless observer.

Life works the same way. God put you in the game on the day you were born with a unique purpose and a role only you can play. He equipped you with the gifts, talents, and potential to make a difference, not just to sit on the sidelines. But here's the thing—it's your responsibility to step up and play to win. No one else can do it for you.

And make no mistake, there's an enemy who knows how valuable you are. Satan's mission is simple: to get you out of the game. If he can trap you in fear and self-doubt, keeping you on the sidelines, he's already won.

His greatest weapon? Fear.

Fear is the ultimate game-changer—not because it's stronger than you, but because it convinces you that you're weaker than you are. It paralyzes you, fills your mind with *"what ifs,"* and whispers lies that you're not good enough.

Fear is the spark that ignites anxiety, setting off a wildfire of worry that's hard to contain. (In the next chapter, we'll dive deeper into this.) Anxiety transforms everyday challenges—like facing Brent Murphy at the plate—into insurmountable obstacles. It magnifies what-ifs, makes problems feel bigger than they are, and leaves you feeling powerless against threats that aren't even real.

But here's the truth: anxiety and fear only win if you let them. You were made to play, not to spectate. The key is not the absence of fear but the presence of courage. And courage isn't the absence of anxiety; it's choosing to step up even when anxiety tries to hold you back.

If only I knew this when I was a kid. I could've experienced the exhilaration of circling the bases on the most feared pitcher in our league!

THE INVITATION

What I didn't know then, that I know now, is that fear is an invitation. You don't have to accept the invitation if you don't want to, but if you do, it's an opportunity to experience peace, confidence, and fulfillment in a way you can't experience otherwise.

Think about it—you cannot have courage apart from fear. If fear doesn't present itself, there's no opportunity to be courageous. You must first feel afraid before you can bust through it and be brave.

Brent's fastball was my invitation to be courageous. Had I faced my fear and stepped up to the plate, chances are something good would have happened. I may not have gotten a hit, but the mere fact of standing in the batter's box would've certainly increased my confidence.

God gave me an opportunity to be courageous as a young boy. I failed, and as a result, I was in absolute turmoil inside. My confidence was crushed, and I left the field that day with no sense of fulfillment.

Where did it all begin? It started when I chose to project fear into the future, turning it into full-blown anxiety that kept me from the very peace I was meant to have.

Decades later, my wife would experience the same thing. And while her anxious thoughts weren't centered on the game of baseball, the crippling effects of projected fear just about caused her to miss the very thing she had been praying for.

I'll let her take it from here.

Tori:

In our book *Beauty in Battle*, I shared my childhood dream of working alongside my husband. But after I got married and as the years passed, that dream felt more like a distant hope. Renowned marriage researcher Dr. John Gottman once said, "At the center of every gridlocked marital conflict is an unrealized life dream."[2] I understood that truth all too well.

As Jason traveled the country, I longed to be more involved in his everyday life. I had grown up watching couples—my parents, grandparents, aunts, uncles, and family friends—work together, and I assumed that was just how marriage worked. I never imagined anything different—until it became my reality. And honestly? I didn't like it.

Then, an opportunity opened. As word spread that Jason had earned his master's degree in counseling, we started welcoming young couples into our home to talk about marriage. What we thought would be a way to encourage others quickly became one of the greatest sources of strength in our relationship. We read every book we could find, and as we sat with these couples, we realized we were learning as much as we were teaching.

That journey led us to write several books together, opening the door to invitations to speak at marriage conferences. And that's when anxiety decided to send its own invitation—one I definitely didn't RSVP for. While Jason wrestled with anxiety before stepping on stage, as he shared earlier, I felt it at just the thought of being up there!

Before our first conference, my body went into full-blown panic mode— cold sores, exhaustion, and a desperate desire to disappear. I finally understood why people rank public speaking as a greater fear than death. And, at the risk of sounding dramatic, it felt like torture.

On the way to the next conference, I got the flu mid-flight. The first night, I was too sick to get out of bed, leaving Jason to cover for me. By morning, I forced myself onto the stage, struggling through every word. Desperate, I begged God to take away the anxiety that consumed me whenever I had to speak publicly.

Fast forward several years, and I was making progress. When we accepted an invitation to speak at an event in Colorado, I noticed a shift—I wasn't overwhelmed by the usual anxiety leading up to the event.

Things were going smoothly ... until we arrived at the venue. As we entered the beautifully decorated ballroom, my eyes locked on renowned author and speaker Dr. Gary Chapman. With his usual enthusiasm, Jason threw an arm around his shoulder and said, "Dr. Chapman, I want you to meet my wife."

Then, as if I wasn't already intimidated enough, he added, "Tor, did you know Dr. Chapman has sold over 20 million copies of *The Five Love Languages*, and it's the bestselling marriage book of all time?"

Dr. Chapman, humble and gracious, simply smiled and turned the conversation back to us. "So, what are you guys speaking on tonight?"

And just like that, a wave of heat rushed over my body. My stomach sank. My mind spiraled: *I can't do this. Who am I to stand on stage and speak to Gary Freaking Chapman? This is Jason's calling, not mine.*

I barely remember the conversation—just the intrusive thoughts that hijacked my confidence.

As soon as we finished talking, I slipped away to the ladies' room. "God, I need You," I whispered, shutting myself into a stall. "I thought I was past this. I hate this feeling. I don't want to be here. Please, talk to me. Help me!"

I stood there, staring at the back of the stall door as if God Himself might be looking back at me. And then, in the stillness, He spoke—not audibly, but unmistakably.

"You don't have to do this," He whispered. "I'm inviting you to do this with Me."

My mind drifted back to the years when Jason was doing so much without me, and my heart ached to be with him. I had prayed many times for God to make a way. Speaking on stage wouldn't have been my first choice, but here we were together. At that moment, my Heavenly Father gently reminded me that He, too, had a dream of us working side by side. Speaking at a conference like this was His invitation to do just that.

Tears slipped down my cheeks. God hadn't called me to prove myself—He had simply invited me to be part of what He was doing. It wasn't about my performance; it was about His presence. He was there, and He had asked me to join Him.

Slowly, my fear of failure gave way to gratitude. Gratitude that the God of the universe had said to me, "Wanna come, Tor?"

Suddenly, Peter's story made perfect sense to me—when Jesus told him to get out of the boat and he walked on water for one brief moment, only to sink in the next.

Just like Peter, I was being invited into something completely outside my nature—something terrifying. And I had two choices: fixate on myself and sink or fix my eyes on the One who said, "Come," and step out onto the water.

My heart shifted. Instead of fear, I felt a surge of excitement. *Yeah, I wanna come!*

I stepped back into the ballroom, still absorbing the weight of God's invitation. As I scanned the faces around me, I realized—God had something for these people tonight, and He had invited me to be part of it.

The thought of "I *have* to do this" faded into "I *get* to do this."

And instead of agonizing over what I had to offer, I started experiencing the joy of simply accepting the invitation.

CHAPTER 2

EXPOSING THE ENEMY

*"Our anxiety does not come from
thinking about the future,
but from wanting to control it."*
–Kahlil Gibran

〜

Now that you know anxiety isn't just something to run from—but an invitation from God to exercise faith over fear and step into His peace—let's take a moment to expose the enemy for what it is. After all, you can't fight a battle if you don't know what—or who—you're up against.

Here's the truth: Anxiety is not your real enemy—Satan is!

I'm guessing you already knew that, but sometimes, we need a reminder. While Satan is the true enemy, anxiety is one of his favorite weapons. It's his way of keeping you distracted, overwhelmed, and stuck in fear instead of walking in faith.

So, for the sake of this chapter, we're going to treat anxiety like the enemy—not because it's the ultimate threat, but because it's the tool the enemy uses to keep you from walking in freedom.

Anxiety is far more than just stress or occasional worry; it's a relentless, intrusive force that takes over your thoughts and emotions. It thrives in uncertainty, fuels fear, and magnifies challenges, making even the smallest problems feel overwhelming and impossible to overcome.

As it takes hold, anxiety begins to distort reality, convincing you that the worst-case scenario isn't just possible—it's inevitable. This creates a cycle of fear where the mere anticipation of danger feels as real as the danger itself. Over time, anxiety traps you in a constant state of survival mode, robbing you of peace and preventing you from fully living.

A quote I recently read captures this beautifully:

"The anticipation of loss is much more frightening than the actual loss as anticipation leaves room for the imagination to create that which, in all likelihood, will never transpire."[3]

Anxiety is not about the pain, but the fear that pain is coming. It's not the size of the bear in the woods but the suspicion that one is there.

Max Lucado summarizes the anxious mindset beautifully in his book, *Anxious For Nothing*.

"Fear sees a threat. Anxiety imagines one. Fear screams, '*Get out!*' Anxiety ponders, '*What if?*' Fear creates fight or flight. Anxiety creates doom and gloom. Fear is what you feel when you see a snake in the yard. Anxiety is what you feel when you decide to never walk across your lawn again."[4]

I'll say this more than once in these pages—I'm not a doctor, psychiatrist, or anxiety expert with all the answers. I'm just a stubborn former jock who thought I had life figured out until anxiety came along, knocked me flat, and forced me to sit still long enough to think about how I was going to fight back.

My goal in defining anxiety is not to give you a lengthy medical breakdown filled with technical jargon. Instead, I want to share the definition that helped me finally see it for what it really is—a deceptive, overblown bully that thrives in the dark. Once you shine a light on it, you can expose it, understand it, and—most importantly—take back control.

THE PROJECTION

Anxiety, in its simplest form, is projected powerlessness.

Anxiety peers into the future and pictures something bad or negative happening that we cannot control. The mind imagines disaster, and the body responds as if it's already happening—heart racing, palms sweating, dizziness, tunnel vision, and a full-body sense of dread.

As we saw in the introduction, anxiety uses fear to its advantage. The night our alarm went off, we were 100% convinced we were about to meet our end. Even after realizing it was a false alarm, our bodies didn't get the memo right away—it took a while for the panic to wear off and for reality to sink in.

Fear is tied to a past or present threat. Anxiety, on the other hand, is about a future threat. It takes what *might* happen and convinces us it *will* happen, filling the unknown with fear and worst-case scenarios.

In the days and weeks after that infamous false alarm, our kids wanted nothing to do with their bedrooms. They were terrified. No matter how many times we reassured them that they were safe and that no one had truly broken in, their little minds were hijacked by anxiety. Their thoughts spun out of control, obsessing over the *possibility* of it happening again, and more than that, how powerless they felt to stop it.

That's the real danger of anxiety—it isn't just about fear. It's about the fear of losing control. Anxiety doesn't just project fear into the future—it *projects powerlessness.*

This is why the Bible is filled with verses reminding us to trust God, put our faith in Him, and refuse to be ruled by fear. Scripture makes it clear—we have an enemy set on our destruction, and fear is one of his favorite weapons. But the Bible is also packed with powerful stories of people who stood their ground in the face of overwhelming fear— moments where anxiety could have easily taken over. Instead, they chose faith. And every single time, God showed up and proved Himself faithful.

Moses stood before the Red Sea with an army closing in behind him; he trusted God, and the waters parted.

Daniel was thrown into a den of lions for refusing to stop praying, but God shut the lions' mouths.

Shadrach, Meshach, and Abednego faced execution in a fiery furnace, yet they refused to bow to fear—and God met them in the fire.

Esther risked her life to save her people, choosing faith over fear despite the danger before her, and God came through.

Each of these stories reminds us that faith is the antidote to fear. The key isn't trying to control everything; it's trusting God with what we can't control and refusing to let anxiety take the wheel. When we place our trust in Him, He doesn't just take away our fear—He steps in and moves powerfully, reminding us that He is always in control.

In Part Two, we'll explore three practical steps to living out this kind of faith—the kind that breaks anxiety's grip, brings real peace, and leads you into true rest. Until then, remember this:

Faith projects power into the future—not because it knows every outcome but because it trusts the One who does.

"Faith is how we handle what we can't see" (Hebrews 11:2).[5]

Fortunately, the Bible doesn't sugarcoat the struggles of even the greatest heroes of our faith. Over and over, we see them battling fear and anxiety, sometimes giving in to panic instead of trusting God— letting worry take over and giving the enemy an opening to wreak havoc in their lives.

Abraham lied about Sarah being his wife *twice* because he feared being killed by powerful rulers.

Moses argued with God at the burning bush, convinced he wasn't good enough for the task.

The Israelites, after witnessing miracle after miracle, still panicked in the wilderness, constantly doubting God's provision.

The boldest prophet in the Bible—Elijah—stood fearlessly against 450 false prophets and called down fire from heaven. But when Queen Jezebel threatened to kill him, he ran for his life and fell into deep despair.

But the most powerful story—the one that will serve as the foundation for everything we'll unpack moving forward—is what happened to the disciples in a boat on a storm-swept sea, as told in Matthew 8:23-27.

This story gives us a front-row seat to see anxiety at work, convincing these Jesus followers to project powerlessness into the future and spiral into fear, even with Jesus right there beside them.

WHO'S IN YOUR BOAT?

One day, Jesus instructed His disciples to get into a boat and cross to the other side of the sea. It wasn't a suggestion but a directive from the Son of God Himself. As they set out, Jesus, fully at peace, fell asleep in the stern. Then, out of nowhere, a massive storm hit—the kind of storm that makes even seasoned fishermen panic.

And panic, they did.

Instead of anchoring themselves in what they knew to be true, the disciples projected fear into the future, imagining the worst possible outcome. Despite being men who had spent their lives on the water and had weathered many storms before, this time was different. Why? Because anxiety took over, hijacking their ability to think clearly and trust that Jesus' word was enough.

Instead of recalling that Jesus had sent them into the boat with a purpose, they fixated on the storm. Instead of trusting in His presence, they convinced themselves that death was inevitable. Instead of remembering that the Messiah—the very one who had performed miracles before their eyes—was right there with them, they let their fear reshape reality.

They woke Jesus in pure panic, shouting, *"Lord, save us! We're going to drown!"* (Matthew 8:25).

Notice their words—"We're *going to* drown!" They pictured themselves in the water, descending uncontrollably to their death. They projected powerlessness into the future, assuming the worst without any evidence beyond the storm in front of them.

But here's the key: Jesus was in the boat the entire time. The One who created the very waters they feared was sleeping through the storm, unshaken.

And yet, how did He respond when they woke Him?

"'You of little faith, why are you so afraid?' Then, He stood up, rebuked the wind and waves, and instantly, everything was calm" (Matthew 8:26).

Jesus wasn't rebuking them for feeling fear—He was rebuking them for letting fear overcome their faith. They required Him to calm the storm *outside* before they could find peace *inside*. But faith doesn't wait for external circumstances to settle. Faith declares peace even in the middle of the storm.

So, what should the disciples have done? Instead of reacting out of fear, they should have responded with faith. Instead of assuming their destruction, they should have anchored themselves in the fact that Jesus Himself had sent them out onto that water. If He said they were going to the other side, nothing—not the wind, the waves, or the storm itself—could stop them from getting there.

Imagine if Jesus had woken up to find them rebuking the wind and waves themselves, standing firm in faith instead of shrinking in fear. Instead of saying, "You of little faith," maybe He would have smiled and said, "Now that's the kind of trust I desire."

But that's not how it played out. Instead, we get an incredible story that reminds us that even our greatest heroes wrestled with fear and anxiety. Their struggle proves that we're not alone in this battle.

A WORD FROM PETE

Living by faith over fear wasn't an easy lesson for Peter—Christ's boldest and most impulsive disciple. Refusing to project powerlessness into the future didn't come naturally to him. He was right there in the boat that day when the storm hit, convinced he was about to die. (Knowing his personality, he might have been the one who suggested waking Jesus up in the first place.)

I can only imagine how much he replayed that moment in his mind afterward, determined not to repeat the same mistake. But then, sometime later—we don't know exactly how long—Peter found himself in another boat and caught in another storm. This time, however, Jesus wasn't asleep in the stern. He was walking on the water toward them.

The disciples, already rattled by the storm, thought they saw a ghost. But Peter, now operating in full faith-mode, spoke up:

"Lord, if it is you, command me to come to you on the water."

Jesus simply responded, *"Come"* (Matthew 14:28-29).

And just like that, Peter stepped out of the boat and walked on water toward Jesus.

What incredible faith! He got it right this time—choosing faith over fear instead of panicking like before. He wasn't about to make the same mistake twice. Bravo, Pete! He passed the test!

Well … almost.

Something happened to Peter—something every one of us can relate to. The moment he looked around and fully grasped what he was doing, fear crept in.

"But when he saw the wind, he was afraid, and beginning to sink, he cried out, 'Lord, save me'" (Matthew 14:30).

The trauma from his last stormy boat ride overpowered his trust in the One who had control over it all. Instead of projecting faith forward, he projected fear, imagining his inevitable downfall the second he started to sink.

How did this happen? How did he shift from faith-mode to fear-mode in an instant?

He took his eyes off Jesus. The object of his fear replaced the object of his faith. The wind. The waves. The overwhelming reality of where he was standing. And in that split second, anxiety grabbed the controls and launched him into full-blown panic.

Look how Jesus responded:

"Jesus immediately reached out his hand and took hold of him, saying to him, 'O you of little faith, why did you doubt?'" (Matthew 14:31).

Same rebuke, different story. And honestly, haven't we all been there? I know I have, so no judgment toward Pete.

But here's the interesting part: When Jesus asked, *"Why did you doubt?"* who was Peter doubting? It wasn't Jesus. He knew Jesus could walk on water; he was watching Him do it.

Peter wasn't doubting who Jesus was—he was doubting who he was. He didn't question Jesus' power; he questioned his own. At that moment, he stopped believing he could be like Jesus. That's when anxiety took over. That's when fear spiraled out of control. And that's when he started to sink—not because Jesus left him, but because he lost confidence in his ability to stand firm in what Jesus had empowered him to do.

Fortunately, Jesus was patient with Peter, just like He is with us. When we let fear overtake our faith and start sinking, He's always there, ready to pull us back up.

What happened to Peter is exactly what happens to us. It's how anxiety pulls the alarm and uses fear to send us into a panic. The moment Peter took his eyes off Jesus and fixated on the chaos around him, anxiety seized control and convinced him he was going to drown.

But here's the truth: the alarm wasn't pulled by reality; it was pulled by anxiety. The reality was that Jesus had called Peter out of the boat, which meant he had nothing to fear. No matter how fierce the wind, how high the waves, or how impossible it seemed, Peter had something greater than the storm itself—he had divine buoyancy. As long as Jesus had given the word, no hurricane wind or wave was strong enough to take him under.

Here's the best part: about 30 years later, long after Jesus had ascended into heaven and Peter had become the leader of the fastest-growing movement in world history—the church—he wrote a letter to persecuted Christians in Asia Minor. In it, he shared a piece of wisdom that still hits home today:

"Be alert and of sober mind. Your enemy the devil prowls around like a roaring lion looking for someone to devour" (1 Peter 5:8).

Peter got to the heart of the issue in one powerful sentence. He called out the real enemy—the devil—and pinpointed exactly where the battle occurs: in our minds. Peter had learned firsthand what happens when anxiety takes over, and decades later, he passed down a hard-earned lesson—staying clear-headed and grounded in truth is the key to standing firm against fear (we'll get to the practicals later).

But here's the thing about lions—they may be powerful, but not invincible. Satan is all roar but no bite. Anxiety may come prowling, trying to intimidate you, but you don't have to run, hide, or play dead. You've got something far stronger: the truth of God's Word, the power of the Holy Spirit, and the authority to tell that overgrown house cat to get lost.

Remember, Jesus is in your boat! No matter what storms come your way, you can trust you'll make it through. Instead of looking ahead with fear and uncertainty, look ahead with confidence, knowing the Son of God is with you. If He's not sinking, neither are you!

So, the next time anxiety tries to sink its claws into you, take a page from Peter's book—stay clear-headed, stand your ground, and remind the enemy he's already been defeated.

Or, you could totally freak out and get a nice little rebuke from Jesus, like the disciples did—but where's the fun in that?

CHAPTER 3

A PEEK UNDER THE HOOD

"Anxiety is like a toddler.
It never stops talking, tells you you're wrong
about everything, and wakes you up at 3 a.m."
–Anonymous

~~~~~~~

Let's take a look at how anxiety works (aka, why your brain freaks out over things that haven't even happened yet).

Quick heads-up—we're about to nerd out on some of the technical stuff behind anxiety. If that sounds about as fun as reading the terms and conditions of a software update, feel free to skip to the next chapter. But hear me out. I've kept it simple because when I was deep in the trenches of anxiety, understanding what was happening in my body helped—a lot. So buckle up (or bail out), but either way, you've been warned.

One of my favorite people to read when it comes to the technical aspects of anxiety is Dr. Archibald Hart.[6] His books and research were a total game-changer for me.

Let's break down how anxiety works in a way that makes sense and doesn't require a medical degree. To do that, we'll use an analogy everyone can relate to—a car.

Here are the key players:

- **Your body** → The car
- **Your brain** → The boss

- **Your nervous system** → The driver
- **Sympathetic nervous system** → The gas pedal
- **Parasympathetic nervous system** → The brake pedal

Think of your body as a high-end luxury car—sleek, powerful, and built for performance. Your brain is the boss, riding in the backseat, calling the shots. But it's not driving the car. That job belongs to your nervous system—the chauffeur—responsible for carrying out the boss's commands and responding to whatever's happening on the road.

Within that nervous system are two key controls: the sympathetic nervous system, which acts like the gas pedal, revving things up when danger is detected; and the parasympathetic nervous system, which works like the brake pedal, slowing things down and restoring calm once the threat has passed.

When everything is working as it should, the driver responds smoothly to the boss's direction—accelerating when necessary, braking when safe, and cruising in balance. This keeps the ride steady and comfortable.

But then anxiety storms into the car—an unwelcome intruder that manipulates through fear to take control. It shoves its way into the backseat and convinces the boss—your brain—that a hitman is tailing you in a blacked-out SUV. Now, instead of calmly navigating the road, the boss starts freaking out, shouting frantic orders, and demanding the driver floor it.

Your nervous system—the poor, panicked driver—has no choice but to obey. If the boss screams, "HIT THE GAS! WE'RE IN DANGER!" the driver slams the gas pedal to the floor, flooding your body with stress signals and launching you into full-blown fight-or-flight mode.

Your body—the car—immediately responds to the chaos. The engine revs high, the tires grip the road, and warning lights flash like something is seriously wrong. Your heart races, your muscles tense like an overworked engine, and suddenly, you're speeding toward panic mode—not because there's a real danger, but because your anxious backseat intruder insists there is.

This is exactly how anxiety hijacks your system. It takes over your brain, floods it with worst-case scenarios, and sends your nervous system into overdrive—forcing it to react as if you're being chased down by danger. Instead of smoothly navigating life's challenges—hitting the gas when needed and tapping the brakes when it's time to slow down—you're stuck in a runaway car, swerving wildly in response to threats that exist only in your imagination.

Let's break down each part of this chain reaction to understand exactly what's happening. The better we know how each player operates, the easier it will be to recognize when anxiety is taking over and, more importantly, how to regain control.

I did my best to keep this as clear and simple as possible, but there's still a lot of information and a few weird words to deal with. So take your time, and don't hesitate to re-read if needed. I have to review tough concepts at least a dozen (or more) times before they finally stick! (Tori: *Does this apply to washing dishes?!*)

YOUR BRAIN

If you grew up in the '80s, you'll remember the iconic commercial where someone holds up an egg and says, "This is your brain." Then they crack it onto a sizzling frying pan—"And this is your brain on drugs."

The same concept applies to your brain on anxiety. Your brain is wired to help you. It's designed to process information, make decisions, and keep you safe. But introducing anxiety into the mix is like throwing that egg straight into the fire—it fries your brain, rewiring it in a way that works against you instead of for you. Just like old-school car thieves hot-wired cars to take control, anxiety hijacks your brain and rewires it to run on fear.

The human brain is wired for survival.[7] This goes back to caveman days when life wasn't about whether or not people liked your Instagram post; it was about not getting eaten by a sabertooth tiger. The brain's job was simple back then: see danger, panic immediately, and run like crazy. This was useful when the threat was real and furry with sharp teeth.

Fast-forward to today, and your brain still uses the same survival playbook, even though the dangers have changed. Instead of tigers lurking in the bushes, we now have work deadlines, financial stress, and the ever-terrifying text that says, "We need to talk."

That's when anxiety storms onto the scene. The moment it takes over, it grabs the control center of your brain, throws logic out the window, and starts screaming "EMERGENCY! EMERGENCY!" on an endless loop. Your nervous system? It's the unlucky hostage in this whole mess, forced to obey anxiety's every irrational demand—whether there's an actual crisis or just a mildly awkward social interaction ahead.

Now, let's look at how this hostage situation unfolds.

YOUR NERVOUS SYSTEM

Your nervous system is your body's communication highway, delivering messages between your brain and the rest of your body.

Your brain is the command center, processing what's happening and making decisions, while your nervous system is the execution team, carrying out orders. It controls everything from muscle movement to internal organ function, ensuring you react appropriately to whatever is happening around you.

In our car analogy, your nervous system is the driver, following orders from the boss (your brain) and deciding when to speed up or slow down based on the situation. It operates through two main divisions: one that revs you up for action by pressing the gas and another that slows you down by pumping the brakes to keep things in balance.

The Sympathetic Nervous System (Gas Pedal)

This is the part of your nervous system responsible for your fight-or-flight response. It puts the pedal to the metal at the first sign of trouble—real or imagined. If you see a bear in the woods? Boom! Sympathetic system activated. If you just *think* about embarrassing yourself during a speech? Boom! Same reaction. Your heart races, your breathing quickens, and your body prepares to either run or throw hands.

The Parasympathetic Nervous System (Brakes)

This is the rest-and-digest part of your nervous system, responsible for calming you down after the perceived threat has passed. Ideally, once the bear leaves (or your speech is over), your parasympathetic system kicks in and presses the brakes, slowing your heart rate and helping you feel normal again. It's the deep sigh of relief and the feeling of peace when you realize your worst-case scenario *didn't* actually happen.

The problem? When anxiety seizes control of the brain's command center, it tricks the driver (your nervous system) into flooring the gas and refusing to hit the brakes, leaving you stuck in a constant state of high alert. Your brain keeps firing off false alarm signals, convincing your body that danger is everywhere, even when nothing is truly wrong. And since your parasympathetic system—the part responsible for slowing things down—fails to kick in properly (because of anxiety), you're caught in an endless loop of tension, overthinking, and exhaustion, running on fumes with no way to pull over.

So, if you've ever felt like your body refuses to relax—like you're stuck in stress mode even when everything is fine—you can thank your overworked sympathetic system and a parasympathetic system that's too tired to slow things down.[8] Thank you, Anxiety.

This is why renewing our minds in God's Word is so important. If we're not consistently feeding our brains truth, anxiety will gladly take over and hold our nervous system hostage, keeping the gas pedal floored until we run out of gas. We'll discuss how to stop this from happening in Part Two of this book.

HORMONES

So, where do hormones come into play? Just as the brain directs the nervous system, the sympathetic system signals hormones to jump into action, ensuring the body's response to stress.

Hormones are tiny chemical messengers that the sympathetic nervous system dispatches throughout the body. They deliver important instructions to the organs and keep everything running smoothly.

Feeling hungry? That's a hormone. Feeling sleepy? Another hormone. Suddenly filled with rage because someone put the cereal box back empty? Yep, hormones again. They control everything from your mood to your energy levels, and when it comes to anxiety, two of them take center stage: adrenaline and cortisol—your body's emergency response team.

The second your nervous system detects something happening—whether it's a real emergency or you realize you forgot to reply to a work email from three days ago—it sends a distress signal to its sympathetic department. This department immediately slams the gas pedal to the floor by firing off adrenaline and cortisol to handle the "emergency."[9]

Adrenaline is the first to show up. It floods your system in seconds, pumping up your heart rate, increasing blood flow to your muscles, and making you feel ready to fight, run, or—if you're like most of us—stand there awkwardly, questioning your life choices. That's why your hands get clammy, your chest tightens, and your vision goes wonky—your body thinks you're facing a bear when you're just trying to answer an email.

Cortisol is the more strategic (but equally dramatic) hormone. While adrenaline is all about immediate response, cortisol is the long-term stress manager. It keeps you alert and on edge long after the initial surge of adrenaline fades. It's also responsible for making sure your body has enough energy to sustain stress, so it messes with digestion, slows down unnecessary functions (like, you know, relaxation), and keeps you awake at 2 AM, replaying that embarrassing thing you said five years ago.

Adrenaline slams the gas pedal to the floor, launching you into full-blown panic, while cortisol acts like the car's cruise control—holding it down so the panic keeps going. That's helpful if you're running from real danger, but not so much when the "threat" is nothing more than a meeting with your boss.

Once the "danger" has passed—or at least once your brain decides to chill—the parasympathetic nervous system calmly presses the brakes. This system tells your body:

- "Okay, false alarm. Let's dial everything back."
- Heart rate? Lower it.
- Breathing? Slow it down.
- Tension? Let's relax those muscles.
- Adrenaline and cortisol? Time to flush them out.

Ideally, the parasympathetic system is like a wise old mentor in an action movie—the one who steps in after the chaos, puts a hand on your shoulder, and says, "Breathe. It's over. You're safe now." It slows your heart rate, relaxes your muscles, and brings your body back to baseline, restoring a sense of calm after your nervous system's unnecessary overreaction.

Here's where things go off the rails—when anxiety takes over the control center of your brain and stays in charge, your sympathetic nervous system stays on high alert while your parasympathetic nervous system struggles to bring things back to normal. Instead of settling down once the stress has passed, your body keeps producing cortisol, leaving you in a constant state of stress.

Over time, this constant cycle of stress hormones messes with everything:

- Your sleep (because your body still thinks it needs to stay alert).
- Your digestion (because cortisol slows it down to "save energy").
- Your immune system (because stress takes priority over fighting off that cold you've had for three weeks).
- Your mood and memory (because too much cortisol shrinks the part of your brain responsible for emotional regulation and clear thinking).[10]

Long story short? When your nervous system overuses adrenaline and cortisol, everyday stress feels like life or death, leaving you stuck in a loop of tension, worry, and exhaustion.

Understanding this is key because once you know how your body operates, you can start retraining it to calm down when it should—to let off the gas and pump the brakes. But we'll get to that later. For now, just remember this: your nervous system is only following orders from your brain. And if anxiety has seized control of your thoughts, it will convince you that every little thing is a life-threatening emergency when, in reality, it was just an email … or an awkward pause in a conversation.

You don't have to let anxiety call the shots. You can learn to break the cycle, calm your nervous system, and take back your peace.

And next time your brain starts screaming, "We're all gonna die!" just remind it:

"Relax, buddy. We're just giving a speech, not running from a tiger."

CHAPTER 4

THREE DAMAGING EFFECTS

"Man is not worried by real problems
so much as his imagined anxieties
about real problems."
–Epictetus

We've defined anxiety as projected powerlessness and explored how it works—now it's time to examine its damaging effects. Anxiety isn't just a feeling or sensation that comes and goes; it's a powerful force that seeps into every part of your life. Left unchecked, it distorts your perspective and drains your energy, holding you back from becoming the person God created you to be.

In this chapter, we'll break down how anxiety takes hold.

Simply put, anxiety does three things:

- It hijacks your brain.
- It distorts your emotions.
- It perverts pressure.

Anxiety Hijacks Your Brain: It's the unwelcome intruder that barges in and screams threats in an attempt to seize control of your mind. It overrides rational thinking, shifting your brain into survival mode, where fear becomes the loudest voice in the room. Instead of responding with clarity or faith, you react out of panic.

Anxiety Distorts Your Emotions: God designed emotions to move us toward action, but anxiety twists them into sources of fear and paralysis. Instead of serving as helpful signals, they become overwhelming and misleading, convincing us that danger is imminent.

Anxiety Perverts Pressure: Pressure itself isn't inherently bad; it can be a tool for growth and motivation. But anxiety distorts it, turning healthy challenges into unbearable burdens. Instead of seeing pressure as an opportunity to trust God and grow stronger, anxiety makes us feel like we are doomed to fail, leading to stress, burnout, or even panic.

Let's look at each of these individually.

THE HIJACK

I'm unsure why, but I've always been drawn to thrillers with hijack situations. There's something about watching the bad guys take over a plane or train and the good guys fight to get it back that keeps me hooked. Turns out, it's the perfect picture of what happens when anxiety hijacks our brain—and what we can do to take it back.

To hijack something means to take it over and use it for a different purpose.[11] That's exactly what anxiety does—it takes over your thoughts and reshapes how you see the world.

My dad used to say, "The warfare for your soul takes place on the battleground of your mind." He was right. The fight against anxiety starts in your thoughts—because what takes hold in your mind shapes everything else.

The movie *Inside Out 2* perfectly illustrates how the battle against anxiety starts in the mind. The film brings emotions to life inside the mind of 11-year-old Riley, showing how Joy, Sadness, Anger, Fear, and Disgust work together to shape her thoughts, decisions, and memories.

Then, Anxiety shows up. At first, it seems helpful—planning ahead, preparing for what might go wrong, and trying to protect Riley from failure. But it quickly becomes clear that Anxiety isn't interested in being part of the team. It takes over, pushing the other emotions aside, convinced that the only way to stay safe is to control everything.

This is when the hijacking happens. Anxiety seizes Riley's brain, flooding her thoughts with an overwhelming number of *what-if* scenarios. Suddenly, everyday challenges feel like major threats.

Joy, the guiding force that once led Riley's decisions, is shoved into the background, showing how anxiety often silences peace, excitement, and hope in our minds. Anxiety doesn't just suggest caution—it demands control and pulls the alarm.

The movie mirrors how anxiety operates in real life—it overrides rational thinking and fuels a constant state of worry. Anxiety won't settle for a seat at the table; it wants to run the whole show, taking the primary position in our minds. It believes that eliminating uncertainty can eliminate all risks, but in doing so, it robs us of the ability to experience life fully.

Just like in the movie, when anxiety seizes control, it shuts out other essential emotions, making it nearly impossible to experience true joy and peace. Left unchecked, anxiety will dominate your thoughts and leave you a shell of the person God made you to be.

But it doesn't have to be that way. Just like Riley, you're not powerless against anxiety's grip. You can take back control of your mind. After all, "... *we have the mind of Christ!*" (1 Corinthians 2:16)

But we're getting ahead of ourselves. We'll get to the way you take back control in Part Two. Before we get there, let's take a deeper look at how anxiety distorts emotions.

THE DISTORTION

Anxiety doesn't only hijack your brain—it messes with your emotions, too. It takes normal feelings and twists them into overwhelming waves of dread and uncertainty. It tricks you into believing that whatever you *feel* must be *true*, making you react to imagined dangers as if they were real.

God wired us as emotional beings. We're made in His image. Emotions are not just a human trait—they are a reflection of the very nature of God. Have you ever considered that God experiences the same emotions we do? According to the Bible, God expresses love, anger, compassion, joy, sorrow, jealousy, and even hatred toward sin and injustice. These emotions are not random or meaningless; they serve a purpose in God's nature and ours.

God designed emotions to be more than just feelings; they are catalysts for action. He wired them into our DNA because an emotion is *an impulse to act*. They are built-in motivators that push us toward a response.

When we feel something deeply, it compels us to act. Love moves us to serve, anger moves us to confront injustice, sorrow moves us to seek comfort, and joy moves us to celebrate. (Maybe God watched *Inside Out* before He created us??!!)

Jesus Himself displayed a full range of emotions—He wept at the loss of a friend, showed righteous anger at corruption in the temple, felt deep compassion for the hurting, and expressed overwhelming joy in God's plan. If Jesus, the perfect Son of God, experienced emotions without sin, then emotions themselves cannot be bad. The real challenge is what we do with them—whether we let them lead us into wisdom or allow them to drive us into destructive patterns.

Anxiety takes a normal, healthy emotion—like concern—and magnifies it until it becomes debilitating.

A simple worry about an upcoming challenge turns into obsessive overthinking.

A natural fear of failure morphs into avoidance and self-doubt.

A fleeting moment of embarrassment mutates into crippling shame that convinces you never to show your face again.

A reasonable desire to be liked spirals into people-pleasing and social anxiety, making even a casual conversation feel like a high-stakes interrogation.

Before you know it, your emotions aren't guiding you. They're holding you hostage.

Instead of moving us toward productive action, anxiety keeps us stuck. It convinces us that every uncomfortable emotion—fear, sadness, frustration—is a sign that something is wrong with us rather than an opportunity to turn to God. Anxiety takes what God designed to help us and twists it into something that holds us back.

Think of your emotions like a car's dashboard warning lights—they don't control the engine but alert you to what's happening under the hood. When working properly, emotions signal what needs attention—fear prompting caution, sadness revealing loss, or joy pointing to something meaningful. They help us navigate life.

However, when anxiety takes over, it distorts your emotional signals and cranks them up to an unbearable level, making minor concerns feel like full-blown crises. Instead of emotions acting as helpful indicators, they become relentless alarms, blaring at full volume and convincing you that danger lurks around every corner.

Using our car analogy from the previous chapter, imagine the unwelcome intruder rewiring your car so that every time your dashboard warning light flickered on, it triggered flashing strobe lights and blared your horn uncontrollably. It wouldn't take long before you were completely overwhelmed, unable to tell if there was an actual problem or if it was just another false alarm.

That's what happens when anxiety distorts our emotions. The problem isn't the emotions themselves—it's that anxiety scrambles their messages, making it nearly impossible to tell the difference between a real threat and unnecessary panic.

Emotions are a gift from God, meant to enhance our lives, not enslave us. When guided by truth, emotions can be powerful allies, but when left unchecked, they can be destructive forces. The key is to let emotions inform us but not control us.

PRESSURE POINT

Anxiety doesn't just hijack your brain and distort your emotions; it also *perverts pressure.*

Pressure is defined as "a force exerted on something or someone."[12] While it often gets a bad rap, pressure is a good thing. We need a certain level of it in our lives. Without it, we lose motivation and purpose, making us ineffective to ourselves and society.

We've identified three distinct levels of pressure:

- Level One – everyday stuff.
- Level Two – events.
- Level Three – emergencies.

Level One Pressure – God designed us to need a certain level of pressure to keep us moving in the right direction. This is the everyday pressure that pushes us to work, earn a living, and care for ourselves and our families. Like the air pressure in a car's tires, the right amount keeps us moving forward, making us productive and useful. Without it, we're not going anywhere. We're stuck in the driveway, unable to move.

As I sit here and write this chapter, I feel Level One pressure to get this chapter done. You wouldn't be reading this if I didn't experience this slight pressure.

Level Two Pressure – Occasional events like tests, speeches, job interviews, or big games can stir up emotions beyond those we experience daily. These moments are temporary but more intense, forcing us to sharpen our focus, steady our breathing, and regulate our emotions to rise to the challenge and perform at our best.

In two weeks, I have to speak on stage in front of 8,000 people. Even the thought of that elevates my breathing to Level Two!

Level Three Pressure – This level is linked to emergencies—those rare, high-stakes moments that appear out of nowhere and trigger our fight, flight, or freeze response. Like my alarm going off in the middle of the night, these times don't come often, but when they do, they demand immediate action. Anything that would make you call 911—or even consider it—falls into this category.

The night we heard someone break into our house (or so we thought), full-blown Level Three!

Level One Pressure is continual. Level Two is occasional. Level Three is rare.

The problem comes when Levels One and Two feel like Level Three. That's what a panic attack is—your mind, body, and emotions spiral out of control, tricking you into believing you're in a full-blown emergency when, in reality, you're not.

That's how anxiety *perverts* pressure. A perversion happens when something is used in a way that goes against its original design. When used correctly, pressure helps shape us into the people God created us to be. Just like a blacksmith applies pressure to mold metal into a tool with a specific purpose, God uses pressure to refine us and make us stronger for His plan. But anxiety corrupts this process, distorting pressure into something paralyzing instead of productive. Instead of pushing us toward growth, anxiety keeps us stuck in fear, preventing us from experiencing peace and purpose.

That intense moment of panic before my speech in Vidalia was a perfect example of a Level Two pressure moment spiraling into a full-blown Level Three crisis. And the car ride afterward? That was just a regular Level One moment—something minor—getting blown up into another Level Three emergency my body was convinced was life-or-death.

How do Levels One and Two begin to feel like Level Three?

When fear enters the mix.

It starts innocently enough ... you're home on a Saturday, enjoying a relaxing day with your family. Then, you remember that big presentation you have to give at work in two weeks. A small wave of nervousness hits—no big deal. But then worry sneaks in. *What if I forget what to say?* That thought picks up speed. *What if I completely freeze?*

Then your brain kicks into overdrive—*What if they laugh? What if I humiliate myself so badly that it haunts me for years?*

Before you know it, your thoughts have spiraled into a full-blown catastrophe. Your heart pounds while a wave of dizziness washes over you. What started as a simple Level One moment—sitting at home with your family—has escalated into a full-blown Level Three emergency, all without you ever stepping up to deliver the presentation.

There's a scientific reason this happens (hello, adrenaline and cortisol). But at that moment, anxiety has perverted pressure and amplified it beyond what it should have been.

At those times, it's important to remember the promise of Psalm 144:12: God has made us "*corner pillars cut for the structure of the palace.*" A pillar isn't just something that holds up weight; it was crafted for that exact purpose.

In the same way, God designed us to handle pressure. When we stand firm in Him, we don't just survive challenges—we stand strong and unshaken, fulfilling the very purpose we were created for, like a corner pillar in a palace.

In those high-pressure moments, God reveals His strength in us, proving the truth of Philippians 4:13: *"I can do all things through Christ who strengthens me."* But when we let anxiety take over, we step away from the strength God has given us.

Pressure is a privilege, but it's hard to see it that way without God's power. The key is learning to hold onto faith rather than giving in to fear when the pressure elevates.

We'll break down a practical way to handle this later, but for now, keep this in mind: When everyday stress (Level One) or occasional challenges (Level Two) start to feel like a full-blown crisis (Level Three), anxiety has seized control.

But here's the truth: God has already given you the strength to handle the pressure you were meant to face. You were made to be a pillar. Now, step into your strength and stand firm.

Don't let anxiety convince you that you're too weak to carry the weight. That's a lie. And in the next chapter, we'll uncover why it's such a convincing one.

CHAPTER 5

GETTING TO THE ROOT

"There are a thousand hacking at the branches
of evil to one who is striking at the root."
–Henry David Thoreau

Anxiety doesn't appear out of nowhere. It has roots.

Just like a tree's strength depends on what's happening beneath the surface, anxiety is often the result of deeper issues that have taken hold over time. If we only focus on managing the symptoms of anxiety without addressing its root causes, we'll find ourselves stuck in the same cycle of fear and worry. To truly overcome anxiety, we need to dig deeper and uncover what's feeding it so we can uproot it for good.

Another quick reminder: We didn't write this book to conduct a scientific investigation into the causes of anxiety, nor are we practicing psychiatrists. If you have the three letters "P, H, and D" after your name, you might find this chapter a little too simplified—and that's exactly the point. We wrote this for everyday people who need clear, practical insight. That's why we've put together an easy-to-remember acrostic to help you pinpoint the root causes of anxiety without needing a medical degree.

We've broken it down into four key categories that spell **STOP!** When you're trying to figure out what's fueling your anxiety, these are the main areas to check:

- **S** – Sin, self-talk, stress.

- **T** – Trauma (both physical and emotional).

- **O** – Origin (genetic factors and your family history).

- **P** – Products (chemical triggers from food, drugs, medications, etc.).

By understanding these root causes, you'll be able to pinpoint what's driving your anxiety and take steps to address it head-on.

THE 3 S's

Sin

My dad taught me early on that whenever you're going through a trial, you need to determine whether it's something God caused for your growth or something you brought on yourself. The way to find out? Simply ask Him. Then, take the time to listen and let Him reveal the answer.

As you'll see later in the book, conviction and anxiety often feel the same. That's why the first place to check when you're struggling with anxiety is your spirit. Ask yourself: *Have I allowed any sin to creep into my life?* The answer will often be no, but it's always the best and safest place to start.

I remember sitting on a plane getting ready to take off from Charlotte when a wave of anxiety hit me out of nowhere. It was intense, just like the episode I mentioned in the introduction. As panic set in, I began praying, asking God to take it away. In the middle of that prayer, He brought three people to mind—former business connections who had wronged me. I thought I had forgiven them, but as I sat there, I realized I was still holding onto bitterness.

What I assumed was anxiety turned out to be God's conviction, His loving hand pressing on me so I could finally deal with the sin I had buried.

Right then, I repented. I asked God to forgive me and fully released those people to Him, even praying for His blessing over their lives. Almost immediately, something started to shift. It didn't all vanish at once, but the weight began to lift. My body felt the release that came through repentance, and I experienced a deeper peace than I had felt in a long time.

Self-Talk

Negative self-talk has a direct impact on our emotions and mental state, fueling fear and doubt without us even realizing it.

In our book *Beauty In Battle*, we discuss how Satan is our adversary who makes accusations for our agreement. Those accusations come in the form of negative thoughts toward ourselves or others. Our job is to refuse to agree with the accuser, choosing instead to stand in truth and confidence.

Satan loves to fill your mind with doubt. He wants you to doubt your ability to give the speech, pass the exam, finish the workout, close the deal, or even be a good parent. If he can get you to question yourself, he's already gaining ground. And he's so crafty in the way he does it.

Pay close attention to this—in the Bible, God's name is *Yahweh*, which means "I AM." More than just a title, the phrase "I AM" declares that God is the ultimate, self-existent, and sovereign source of all power. His authority, existence, and strength aren't dependent on anyone or anything—He simply IS, and His power is limitless and eternal.

When we use "I AM" and follow it with something negative—like "I am not smart," "I am not good enough," or "I am not sure I can get through this"— we're not just making a casual statement. We're assigning power to those words. And whether we realize it or not, we're misusing God's name in the process. By attaching weakness, failure, or defeat to "I AM," we're taking God's name in vain, not just in speech but in belief.

Taking God's name in vain goes far beyond using it as a curse word. It means misusing and diminishing God's power and identity in our words, actions, and thoughts. What we declare about ourselves matters; if we're not careful, we can reinforce lies instead of standing on God's truth.

So when those negative thoughts creep in, take a page from Dr. James Gills, the only person in the world to complete six Double Ironman Triathlons. And if that wasn't impressive enough, he finished his last one at the age of 59. When asked how he did it, he explained:

"I've learned to talk to myself instead of listening to myself. If I listen to myself, I hear all the reasons why I can't finish the race. I'm too tired, too old, and too sore. But if I talk to myself, I can feed myself with the words of encouragement that I need to keep on moving forward."[13]

Stress

Anxiety isn't only triggered by sin or negative self-talk—one of the biggest culprits is stress.

Chapter Three discussed pressure and how we're built to handle a certain amount. Stress is simply the body's reaction to that pressure—physical, emotional, or mental. It kicks in when challenges arise or worries start stacking up, triggering a chain reaction in your mind and body to help you respond. Stress can be a good thing in small doses—it keeps you focused and motivated. But when it lingers too long or piles up too high, it stops being helpful and starts taking a serious toll on your health and overall well-being.

When stress builds up, it triggers the body's fight-or-flight response, flooding us with adrenaline and cortisol—the same hormones released during moments of real danger. Over time, this keeps us in a heightened state of alertness, making even minor challenges feel overwhelming.

Instead of processing stress and moving forward, we get stuck in a cycle of tension—fueling anxiety and making it harder to find peace.

Think of it this way—an average NFL game lasts just over three hours. There are 60 minutes in each game, but in reality, there are only about 11 minutes of actual "live play."[14] Those 11 minutes are when all the action happens and fans go wild. That means players and fans spend most of the time waiting, resetting, and recovering between plays.

Imagine if you tried to scream nonstop for the entire three-hour game. How would that stress affect you? You'd be passed out on the bleachers before the first quarter was over.

Handling stress works the same way. We aren't designed to be constantly on high alert, jumping from one thing to the next while running on caffeine and energy drinks. That's not sustainable. We need intentional rest to function at our best.

If we let external stressors dictate our pace, we'll burn out before halftime. In a later chapter, we'll dive into practical ways to build rhythms of rest and resilience so stress doesn't take over your life.

TRAUMA

While sin, self-talk, and stress are major contributors to anxiety, there's another factor that runs even deeper—trauma. Unlike everyday stress, which comes and goes, trauma leaves a lasting imprint on the mind and body. It can stem from a single overwhelming event or repeated experiences that shake your sense of safety and stability.

Trauma rewires the brain, making it hypersensitive to perceived threats. This is why people who have experienced trauma often struggle with anxiety—they're not just reacting to the present; they're still feeling the echoes of the past.

For our discussion, I want to focus on two types of trauma—physical and emotional.

In his groundbreaking book on stress, published in the '90s before anxiety became a widely researched topic, Dr. Archibald Hart explained that the deepest form of anxiety often stems from physical trauma. You know exactly what he means if you've ever been T-boned at an intersection. The next time you approach a similar intersection, your body reacts before your mind has time to process it. It's not just a mental battle; your nervous system remembers the danger and goes on high alert, even if there's no real threat.

It takes a long time to overcome this type of trauma. But it can be done. So be patient with yourself.

Emotional trauma often operates in the same way. I once asked my dad, who pastored a church for many years and has a treasure trove of incredible stories, why he had never written a book like many other pastors. His response was a powerful reminder of how deeply emotional wounds can shape us—sometimes for a lifetime.

He said, "I won't write a book because Ma McKenna told me I couldn't write."

Confused, I pressed him for more details. He explained, "Ma McKenna was my 11th-grade English teacher. I wrote a paper once, and when she handed it back, it was covered in red ink. I'll never forget how stupid I felt at that moment—and how small she made me feel with how she critiqued me in class. From that day forward, I knew I wasn't a good writer, so I stopped trying."

More than half a century later, that experience still has a hold on him. He told me that any time he tries to write, he can't get through a single sentence without an overwhelming urge to go back and correct it because he still hears Ma McKenna's voice in his head. And even though he eventually grew to enjoy writing in Bible school, the process remained far more difficult than it should have been—all because of a moment in his teenage years that left a lasting mark.

Think about that—a 76-year-old man still wrestling with the emotional trauma he experienced at 17. That's the power of emotional wounds left unhealed. They don't just fade with time; they take root, shaping how we see ourselves and what we believe we're capable of.

This is why processing emotions verbally with someone you trust is so important. Buried emotions never die. And the longer you hold them in, the heavier they get.

Try this: Hold your phone in your hand and extend your arm straight out in front of you at eye level. Feels light, right? Now, keep holding it there for 15 minutes. Suddenly, that little phone feels like a brick. The weight of your phone isn't determined by how heavy it is, but by how long you hold it.

Emotional trauma is the same way. Find someone you can talk to and let it out so you can let it go.

Trauma doesn't just leave a memory—it leaves an imprint on the brain and the body. When trauma is unresolved, it keeps us stuck in a cycle of fear, reacting to past danger as if it's still happening. Understanding this connection is key to breaking free from anxiety and learning how to retrain both our minds and bodies to respond differently.

ORIGIN

Genetic factors and the dynamics in your family of origin play a huge role in discovering the root cause of anxiety. How you are wired and the environment you grew up in lay the foundation for navigating life. Our default reactions to fear, pressure, and uncertainty were formed long before we were even aware of them.

When it comes to genetics, some people run like a sports car. Others, like an RV. If you're a sports car, your engine can get revved up faster and higher than someone who approaches life in a more methodical and relaxed way. So you'll need to be extra mindful in guarding against anxiety, even more than some of your friends who aren't wired the same way.

The way we were raised also affects how we handle anxiety. From a young age, we absorbed more than just lessons on manners and responsibility; we internalized how our parents and caregivers responded to stress, fear, and uncertainty. If our upbringing was marked by constant tension, criticism, unpredictability, or fear, anxiety can take root before we even realize it.

For example, suppose you had a parent who worried excessively about money, safety, or the future. In that case, you may have subconsciously learned that the world is a dangerous, unpredictable place and that you must always be on high alert.

If you were raised in an environment where mistakes were met with shaming instead of grace, you might struggle with perfectionism, constantly fearing failure or disappointing others.

And if your home life lacked emotional security—whether due to divorce, neglect, or unresolved conflict—you may have developed a deep-seated fear of abandonment or rejection, making relationships a source of stress rather than peace.

Even well-meaning parents can unknowingly pass down anxious tendencies by the way they respond to challenges. The good news is that while our upbringing may explain why we feel anxious, it doesn't have to define us. Recognizing the roots of anxiety in our genetic makeup or our family background is a powerful step toward breaking free from it.

PRODUCTS

Finally, when searching for the root of our anxiety, we need to take a closer look at what we're putting into our bodies.

Many people don't realize that anxiety isn't always just a thought problem; sometimes, it's a body problem. The substances we consume—whether it's alcohol, caffeine, certain medications, marijuana, food dyes, or even processed foods—can trigger or intensify anxiety, making it harder to feel calm and in control.[15]

Caffeine

Take caffeine, for example. While that morning cup of coffee might boost energy, too much caffeine can overstimulate your nervous system, causing jitters, a racing heart, and heightened feelings of panic. If you're already prone to anxiety, caffeine can make it worse by keeping your body in a state of heightened alertness, making it harder to relax and think clearly.

This happened just before my brother, David, and I were scheduled to speak to a large group of students at Liberty University—a few months before the full-blown meltdown I shared in the introduction. Looking back, it was a warning sign, a glimpse of what was coming, like the trailer for a movie you don't want to watch.

David mentioned he wanted a quick coffee just before we went on stage. I told him to get me one, too, but to make sure it was decaf. A few minutes later, he handed me the cup, and I took several big sips, wanting to get something in my system before stepping in front of the crowd.

The next thing I knew, I was standing on stage and my head started spinning. My heart was racing, sweat was pouring down my face, and I could feel panic creeping in. While David was speaking, I quietly walked over and grabbed a chair, pulled it on stage, and sat down, trying to compose myself.

I made it through the talk, but was uncomfortable for most of it. David looked at me as we stepped off stage and asked, "What happened? You looked pale as a ghost." I told him I thought I had a panic attack and had no idea what triggered it. Then it hit me—the coffee. I turned to him and said, "You got me decaf, right?"

He casually replied, "No. They didn't have any."

At that moment, it all made sense. The caffeine on my empty stomach had sent my body into overdrive, and my system couldn't handle it. From that day on, I've completely cut caffeine out of my life—especially before stepping on stage!

We always recommend that anyone struggling with anxiety take a break from caffeine and energy drinks. It's a simple first step, and more often than not, it makes a noticeable difference in how they feel.

Substances

Alcohol is another anxiety inducer, but it works in the opposite way to caffeine. Alcohol is a depressant, which means it initially slows down brain activity and makes you feel relaxed. But once the effects wear off, the nervous system rebounds, often leading to increased anxiety. This is known as "hangxiety"—that anxious, restless feeling you get the morning after drinking. While alcohol might seem like a quick fix for stress, it ultimately makes anxiety worse in the long run by throwing off brain chemistry and sleep patterns.

Then there are substances like marijuana and CBD, often marketed as anxiety relievers but just as likely to make things worse. While some people feel temporary relief, once the effects wear off, anxiety can come back even stronger—leading to a cycle of dependence just to feel normal.

While we don't have the time (or the credentials) to dive into the deeper reasons why these substances lead to anxiety, grab a copy of *The End Of Mental Illness* by Dr. Daniel Amen if you want to explore it deeper. We are big fans of Dr. Amen's work in this area.

The real danger of these substances is that they numb the healthy Level One pressure we need to function. Instead of learning to navigate everyday stress, people end up in a permanent state of "chill," dodging responsibility and avoiding growth. Next thing you know, they're unbothered by everything—including the fact that they have no motivation, no direction, and no job. But hey, "It's all good, man," while they ask you for money.

Like any quick fix, alcohol and marijuana don't address the root cause of anxiety. At best, they offer a temporary escape. At worst, they cover up the problem while creating a dependency that makes true healing even harder.

Food

And let's not forget about the food we eat. Processed foods, excessive sugar, artificial additives, and nutrient deficiencies can all mess with brain function and hormone levels, increasing feelings of stress and anxiety. A diet high in sugar and refined carbs, regardless of how delicious they may taste, causes blood sugar spikes and crashes, leaving you feeling shaky, irritable, and on edge.

Think back to the car analogy in Chapter Two—your body is the car, and food is the fuel that keeps it running. If you're constantly filling the tank with junk, don't be surprised when things start to sputter, stall, and break down. It's like pouring a can of Coke into your gas tank instead of fuel—you're not going anywhere but to the mechanic.

Foods loaded with sugar and artificial ingredients overstimulate your nervous system, making it easier for anxiety to take hold. Ever notice how a sugar rush feels great for a few minutes, but then suddenly you crash, feeling drained and jittery? That's because your body just rode a hormonal rollercoaster, and now it's stuck at the bottom of the hill.

When I was struggling with anxiety, I had to drastically cut back on sugar because it was affecting me much like caffeine did—sending my body into overdrive. During that time, the healthier I ate, the better I felt. It wasn't a magic cure, but it made a noticeable difference.

When you've been hit with a major anxiety attack, the quickest and easiest thing to adjust is what you're putting into your body—and sometimes, that small change can make a big impact.

Medication

Our perspective on medication is aimed at the everyday person battling anxiety, not those with severe psychiatric conditions requiring specialized care. So, let's be clear—we're not making blanket statements. We fully recognize that some cases require medical intervention, and for certain individuals, medication plays a role in their treatment plans.

That said, here's our quick take on medication for the rest of us:

Medicine is meant to treat symptoms, not causes; as such, it's meant to be used temporarily, not permanently. If you want a cure, you have to find the cause. But if you've numbed the symptoms alerting you to a problem, you'll call off the search.

You should read that again.

We're not against medication. It has a place. Used correctly, it can create a momentary state of rest that allows the body to heal. Think of a cast on a broken arm—it doesn't heal the bone but provides the stability needed for healing. Or consider anesthesia in surgery—it numbs the pain so the doctor can do the work necessary to fix what's broken. In the same way, medication can help quiet anxiety's blaring alarm so you can do the real work of recovery. But the medicine itself isn't the healer—God is.

God designed our bodies with an incredible ability to heal. But when we rely on medication as a long-term solution instead of short-term support, we undermine that natural healing process. It's like the testosterone shots so many guys are taking now; once they start, their bodies stop producing it on their own.

The same principle applies here. You can take medication to silence anxiety's alarm, but if you don't address the reason it's going off in the first place, it's like wearing a cast on a broken leg while still doing the thing that broke it.

But here's the key difference between anxiety and a broken bone: unlike a fracture that mends with time, anxiety doesn't heal on its own. It requires our participation. We have to engage in the process actively—partnering with God as we renew our minds and replace lies with truth. That's what Romans 12:2 reminds us:

"... be transformed by the renewing of your mind."

God can and will transform you—He can pull you out of anxiety and lead you into peace—but you have a role to play in the process. Like He provided manna for the Israelites in the wilderness but required them to step outside and gather it, overcoming anxiety works the same way. God provides what we need, but we must actively take hold of it. When we do our part—which we'll break down in Part Two—God steps in and does His.

True healing from anxiety doesn't come from medication—it comes from participation.

Medication has its place, but make no mistake—medicines are a tool, not a cure. It was never meant to be the healer. That role belongs to God alone. Lasting freedom comes when we engage with Him, allowing His truth to rewire our minds and restore our peace.

At the end of the day, getting to the root of anxiety means taking an honest inventory of what's fueling it. That's why the STOP method is so helpful—it's a clear framework to identify what's happening beneath the surface.

The goal isn't to place blame or feel overwhelmed by all the possible causes, but to pinpoint where anxiety is gaining a foothold so you can start addressing it head-on. The more awareness you have, the more power you have to break free.

"So if the Son has set you free, you are free indeed!" (John 8:36)

PART ONE SUMMARY

*"Faith is the only thing I know of
that's stronger than fear."*
–Joyce Meyer

———————

Ever finished reading something and immediately forgotten everything you just read? Same. That's why I want to hit pause and do a quick recap—to ensure all this info isn't flying past you like road signs on a highway.

My goal in Part One wasn't to throw a bunch of words at you, but to help you understand why anxiety does what it does so we can show you how to fight back. So before we dive any deeper, let's lock in the key takeaways.

So far, we've discussed the problem with our internal alarm system and tackled four key questions about anxiety:

- What is it?
- How does it work?
- What are its effects?
- What are its root causes?

We laid the foundation by showing that in our greatest moments of fear—when anxiety tries to take the wheel and send us into a tailspin— God is offering us something greater. Those very moments are His invitation to go deeper with Him. What feels like an obstacle is actually an opportunity, a chance to trust Him in a way we never have before.

WHAT IS IT?

At its core, anxiety is *projected powerlessness*. For the everyday person, this is the simplest way to understand its true nature. Anxiety drags our thoughts into the future, convinces us that the worst is inevitable, and traps us in a cycle of fear and uncertainty. When we project fear onto what's ahead, our perspective becomes distorted, making us feel powerless over things that haven't happened yet.

HOW DOES IT WORK?

When anxiety takes over, it hijacks your brain's control center, tossing logic aside and screaming "EMERGENCY!" Your nervous system becomes the hostage, forced to obey every irrational command. It fires off distress signals to your body, flooding it with adrenaline and cortisol.

- Adrenaline floors it, triggering full-blown panic.
- Cortisol keeps it pinned to the floor, making sure the panic lingers.

The result? Your body locks into crisis mode, reacting to the worst-case scenarios your brain imagined, not ones that actually exist.

WHAT ARE ITS EFFECTS?

Anxiety does three major things:

- **It hijacks your brain**, making you react out of fear instead of faith, keeping you stuck in a spiral of doubt and worst-case scenarios.
- **It distorts your emotions**, twisting them into sources of fear and paralysis, turning normal emotional responses into overwhelming alarms that signal danger.
- **It perverts pressure**, transforming healthy challenges into unbearable burdens. Anxiety causes everyday stress (Level One

pressure) and occasional high-stakes events (Level Two pressure) to feel like crisis moments (Level Three pressure). This distortion triggers panic, making us feel like we've lost control, even when there's no real emergency.

WHAT ARE ITS ROOT CAUSES?

We explored the four main areas where anxiety often takes root, using the **STOP** method as a guide:

- **S: Sin, Self-Talk, and Stress** – Anxiety and conviction can feel similar, so we start by asking God if there's any sin we need to address. We then evaluate our self-talk—are we believing lies from the enemy? Lastly, we check our stress levels (especially our schedules) to see if we're overloading ourselves.

- **T: Trauma** – Whether physical or emotional, past trauma can shape how we respond to stress in the present, robbing us of peace and security.

- **O: Origin** – Our family history and genetic makeup play a role in how we process anxiety. Some are wired like high-performance sports cars, while others are more like steady RVs. If anxiety runs in your family or you grew up in a high-stress home, you may have to work even harder to manage it effectively.

- **P: Products** – What we put into our bodies has a direct impact on anxiety. Alcohol, caffeine, sugar, food dyes, processed foods, and even certain medications can heighten anxiety symptoms. Since our bodies are temples of the Holy Spirit, taking care of what we consume isn't just a vital step in managing anxiety but a key to pleasing God.

Now that we've completed Part One, it's time to shift gears. Knowledge is essential, but without action, nothing changes. That's why we've created a simple, three-step plan to help you break free from anxiety's grip. In Part Two, we'll walk through this process step by step, equipping you with the tools to reclaim your peace and step into the life God has called you to live.

Let's get to work!

PART TWO
THE PLAN

*"The great thing about faith in
God is that it keeps a man undisturbed
in the midst of disturbance."*
–Oswald Chambers

Now comes the fun part—the moment we stop letting anxiety call the shots and start fighting back! We're diving into a powerful, three-step plan to crush anxiety, defeat overwhelm, and conquer the fears that freak you out. No more letting worry dictate your life. No more spinning in cycles of doubt and stress.

Part One laid the foundation—you now understand what anxiety is, how it works, its damaging effects, and why it takes hold. Part Two is where we move from understanding to action. It's time to put a weapon in your hand and show you how to wield it.

Anxiety may have been running the show, but that ends now. You're about to take back your peace, your confidence, and your life.

When anxiety hits and sends our internal alarm into overdrive, we have a choice—we can let fear take control, or we can fight back. And to fight effectively, we need a battle plan. Here's how we do it in three simple steps:

- Recognize
- Renounce
- Replace

STEP ONE: **RECOGNIZE** what's happening and pinpoint the source of your fear. As we've said before, the true source is always Satan. He is your enemy, the one whispering lies and planting fear-filled thoughts about the future. But when you shine the light on him, his power crumbles. Knowing that the battle is spiritual and that fear is a tactic, not truth, empowers you to fight back confidently.

This section will cover Chapters 6-11. We'll begin with two foundational principles that set the stage for true freedom, and then the four key areas where the enemy operates, so you can expose his influence. When you learn to spot the enemy every time he shows up, you'll be equipped to take pivotal Step Two.

STEP TWO: **RENOUNCE** the lie you're tempted to believe in the moment of anxiety. Behind every anxious thought is a deception designed to shake your faith. Satan isn't just a liar; he's *the father of lies*. And the most effective lies are the ones that are *almost* true. He knows how to twist reality just enough to make you take the bait, filling your mind with accusations and worst-case scenarios. But here's the key: an accusation only has power if you *agree* with it.

To renounce something means to formally declare your rejection of it—to abandon it and refuse to let it have power over you.[16] This section covers Chapters 12-16, where we will uncover five key lies you must formally reject. Refusing to believe these lies strips them of their influence and prepares us for the third—and most powerful—step.

STEP THREE: **REPLACE** the lie with God's truth. It's not enough to reject the enemy's voice—we must fill that space with the truth that sets us free. Jesus warned in Matthew 12 that when an evil spirit leaves a person, the situation can become even worse if nothing takes its place. The same principle applies to our thoughts. If we don't intentionally replace fear-driven lies with the promises of God, anxiety will creep right back in. Truth is the key that unlocks lasting peace.

We're going all-in on truth in this section—because it deserves that kind of focus. You'll notice we've packed in twice as many chapters as the previous two sections. Why? Because truth doesn't just expose lies—it replaces them with power.

This section includes Chapters 17–26, and in them, we'll unpack ten truth bombs to break anxiety's grip and lead you into real freedom. Think of each one like a divine light switch—a simple shift you can flip in the heat of the moment that will flood your mind with the peace God promises.

This three-step process—**Recognize, Renounce, Replace**—is our battle plan for breaking free from anxiety's grip. And in the chapters ahead, we'll unpack each of these steps in detail, giving you the tools to regain control from anxiety once and for all.

We will break each of these steps into bite-sized, practical principles to help you pinpoint your anxiety and pull it out at the root.

So buckle up—your breakthrough is closer than you think.

Real freedom starts now.

STEP ONE

RECOGNIZE WHAT'S HAPPENING

CHAPTER 6

RECOGNIZE YOUR ENEMY

"No weapon against you shall prosper!"
–Isaiah 54:17

~~~~~~~~

As we laid out in Part One, anxiety begins with the hijacking of your brain. The rest of our time together will be spent exposing the hijacker and the steps we must take to keep him from taking over!

We identified our enemy in Chapter Two, but now it's time to recognize him when he makes his move. You can know everything about how he operates, but if you don't spot him in real-time—right when he strikes—you'll never be able to take him down.

The key is realizing that the battle against anxiety isn't just mental, emotional, or physical—it's ultimately spiritual. And once you recognize that, you can see the enemy clearly for what he is. Think of it like switching to night vision goggles in the middle of a dark battlefield—suddenly, the enemy hiding in the shadows is exposed, and you can take aim with precision.

Anxiety might show up in your body, mind, and emotions, but you'll never truly defeat it if you only fight on those fronts. You have to see the battle as spiritual warfare so you can fight with the right weapons and win. As the prophet Zechariah reminds us:

"… Not by might nor by power, but by my Spirit, 'says the Lord Almighty'" (Zechariah 4:6).

When you truly recognize the enemy, you'll discover one of the most potent truths you need to overcome anxiety—*the thing you fear has no real power over you!* The only power it has is the power you give it.

This principle is perfectly portrayed in *The Wizard of Oz*. I watched it as a kid, and let me tell you, that movie rattled me. The Witch? Terrifying. The Wizard? Just as bad. To an 8-year-old, they were the ultimate nightmare fuel. Luckily, I was a twin and never had to sleep alone. (Tori: *Uh, you still don't sleep alone!*)

The story follows Dorothy, who gets swept away from her home in Kansas and lands in the magical land of Oz, stuck with no way to return. Her one mission? Find her way home. Along the way, she gains a few unexpected travel companions—a scarecrow, a tin man, and a cowardly lion. But she also faces a major obstacle: the Wicked Witch of the West, who's determined to stop her before she can reach the mysterious Wizard of Oz.

The Witch? She's all green skin, with a long nose and that scratchy voice that makes the hair on your neck stand up. And let's not even talk about her flying monkey men. Those little guys haunted me for a good while. The Witch is entirely against Dorothy, and for a good reason—Dorothy has something powerful: her ruby slippers. Dorothy doesn't realize that those slippers hold the key to getting her home. But the Witch knows, and she'll do anything to take them from her.

Then there's the Wizard. When Dorothy finally reaches the Emerald City, she meets this giant, floating head surrounded by smoke and fire. He shouts commands in a voice that shakes the room, making Dorothy and her friends believe he holds the ultimate power.

But here's where it gets good—Dorothy eventually discovers that these terrifying figures aren't so terrifying after all.

The Witch? Turns out, she's desperately afraid of water. In a frantic moment to save her friend, Dorothy tosses a bucket of water to extinguish a fire, and some splashes on the Witch. Next thing you know, she's melting into the floor, screeching, "I'm melting! I'm melting!" Just like that, her biggest enemy is gone.

And the Wizard? When Dorothy and her crew finally stand before him, he's still playing up his whole "Great and Powerful Oz" act. But then Dorothy's little dog, Toto, pulls back a curtain, revealing an ordinary man frantically pulling levers, pressing buttons, and speaking into a megaphone. The giant, fearsome Wizard was a small, regular dude using smoke and mirrors to scare people into submission.

The lesson here? Recognizing your enemy is step one in overcoming him.

Dorothy saw the truth—water was the Witch's weakness, and the Wizard was an illusion. The moment she recognized them for what they truly were, she had power over them.

For our purposes, the Witch represents Satan, while the Wizard represents anxiety.

Satan is your real enemy. He stands against everything you stand for, desperately trying to rob you of the power you already have in Christ. But just like the Witch was powerless against a simple splash of water, Satan is powerless against the living water of the Holy Spirit.

Jesus said:

"Whoever believes in me, as Scripture has said, 'Out of his heart will flow rivers of living water'" (John 7:38).

Satan is terrified of the living water inside you because he knows how the story ends—one day, that water will be the thing that finally takes him out for good. He'll melt like the Witch, but in the eternal Lake of Fire.

That's why, in the meantime, he's working overtime to rob you of your power, doing everything he can to keep you afraid.

The Wizard, on the other hand, represents anxiety—the booming, intimidating voice that makes you feel like you're in danger when you're not. It yells, threatens, and demands your attention, all while hiding behind a curtain, pulling levers to keep you on edge. But when you pull that curtain back—when you *recognize* anxiety for the lie it is—you realize there was nothing to be afraid of.

Dorothy wanted to return home because "there's no place like home." Home represents peace, rest, and fulfillment. And that's what Satan wants to keep you from.

But like Dorothy, once you *recognize* the enemy and expose his tactic of fear-based anxiety as a fraud, you can begin the journey to freedom. You can begin your journey home—to the perfect peace and rest that is found close to the heart of a loving Father.

Turns out, I'm not the only one haunted by those little monkey men in the movie. Tori had her run-in with one of those little demons, too, but hers wasn't a fictional character at all.

TORI'S STORY

Tori:

It happened just after we brought our youngest daughter, Lundi, home from the hospital. I was running on no sleep, operating in full "newborn mom" mode, and constantly waking up in the middle of the night to nurse her. One night, as I sat feeding Lundi in the stillness of the dark, something strange happened.

I saw it.

A shadowy figure appeared at the edge of the bed. It looked like a troll—small, creepy, and unmistakably demonic. It didn't say a word. It didn't need to. Its presence alone was enough to freeze me with fear.

I'm not one of those people who see stuff like this. People like that always freak me out, if I'm honest. So, to say it was a shocking—and terrifying—moment for me is an understatement.

Night after night, it kept happening. I would wake up to nurse, and the figure would be there. Every time it showed up, my heart would race, my thoughts would spiral, and sleep became nearly impossible. It was spiritual warfare showing up in my bedroom, and it was relentless.

A few weeks later, one of Jason's spiritual mentors, Rusty Thomas, came into town and stopped by our house for a visit. Jason told me I should tell him about what was happening and that if anyone could help me, he was the guy.

So I told him about it, expecting a confused look or a polite nod. But without hesitation, he said, "Oh, yeah. I've seen it too. That's a spirit of fear."

I was relieved that he didn't think I was crazy, but I was even more thankful that he knew what I was talking about and had experienced it firsthand.

"You're dealing with spiritual warfare," he explained. "This is Satan trying to disrupt your sleep and steal your peace. But you know he has no power over you, right?"

"Well, I'm losing a lot of sleep each night," I said. "And I'm terrified every time he shows up, so he's feeling pretty powerful right now."

"I get it!" Rusty laughed. "But here's the truth—the only power that thing has is the power you give it through fear. The way you beat it is to stand firm in your authority in Christ and speak to it—out loud.

Declare that you're not afraid because it has no power over you. That's how you shut it down."

But I am afraid, I thought to myself.

"Even if you don't fully believe it at first," he continued. "You speak it until your heart catches up with what you're declaring."

Made sense. So, that's what I decided to do. And like clockwork, the very next night, it showed up again. Remembering Rusty's advice, I looked straight at it, knowing my fear was the only thing feeding it, and said, "I'm not afraid of you."

I said it more than once, just to make sure it got the message.

And full transparency? I was still scared out of my mind. But I spoke it anyway. I *wanted* to believe what I was saying, but I was having trouble truly believing it.

But I didn't stop. And neither did this little guy. He showed up a few times a week for several months, and each time he appeared, I'd say the same thing over and over—"I'm not afraid of you. "

Then, finally, one night, something changed.

It appeared again, just like before, but something inside me was different. I was fed up with letting my fear keep me down. This time, I didn't just say I wasn't afraid—I truly *believed* it. I felt zero fear.

With full conviction, I clenched my fists, gritted my teeth, and declared from the bottom of my soul, "I'M NOT AFRAID OF YOU!!!!!"

And just like that, it disappeared. For good.

It never came back.

God opened my eyes to the spiritual battle we often cannot see and how my fear fuels the enemy's power. The demon only showed up because my fear gave it access. And although it took some time for me to get there, once I truly believed it had no power, it lost its grip.

We're going to dive deeper into the power of belief in Chapter Ten, but for now, I want to give you a verse that reveals something about the powerful combination of confession and belief. This verse shows us how to find salvation for our souls:

"... *If you confess with your mouth that Jesus is Lord and believe in your heart that God raised Him from the grave, you will be saved*" (Romans 10:9).

This is the amazing force of confession and belief. And if that truth has the power to save our souls, it absolutely has the power to break the chains of fear. I had to confess that I was not afraid until I believed it.

God made it clear to me: you often have to speak the truth before your heart fully believes it. It takes time. I had to declare it again and again— out loud—until my brain caught up and my heart aligned.

Because the enemy doesn't flee when you *feel* bold; he flees when you stand in truth. And sometimes that starts with shaky words, whispered in the dark, until your spirit rises and takes its rightful place.

Plenty of situations in life *feel* scary—and some genuinely are. But even then, fear doesn't get to lead unless you let it. Opening your eyes to the spiritual battle that's taking place equips you to fight and win.

I've since learned to apply this lesson in other areas of my life. Not long after seeing the demon at the end of my bed vanish for good, I had an acquaintance who repeatedly crossed personal boundaries. Just the *thought* of that person coming around would stir up the same kind of fear and anxiety.

Instead of letting it take over, I went back to what I learned from the shadowy figure in my bedroom. I spoke truth, reminded myself I wasn't powerless, and put up healthy boundaries—*without fear*. And my anxiety went away. (We'll talk more about boundaries in Chapter 22.)

Fear only has power when you give it authority. When you refuse to give it authority, it has to go.

It reminds me of an old hymn I grew up singing:

"Because He lives, I can face tomorrow. Because He lives, all fear is gone."

It's not just a comforting lyric. It's a spiritual reality. The enemy's threats are empty when you're filled with the living water of the Holy Spirit. Satan only thrives in the shadows, and fear is the flashlight he uses to make them look bigger than they are.

So if you feel like anxiety has been showing up night after night, just like that little troll did—don't shrink back. Speak up. Declare the truth of who you are and the power you have in Christ.

Say it out loud. Say it boldly.

Even if your voice shakes.

Even if you don't fully believe it yet.

Say it anyway. Say it until your heart catches up.

Because when it does, the enemy won't stand a chance.

And—just like the Wicked Witch in Oz—when exposed to the Living Water, he'll melt. He'll vanish. Powerless. Exposed. And completely defeated.

CHAPTER 7

RECOGNIZE YOUR HOPE

"Hope is the dream of the waking man!"
–Aristotle

———————

Forgive me for another movie reference, but there's a moment in *A Charlie Brown Christmas* that's easy to miss—yet incredibly powerful when you see it. Linus, who is practically glued to his trusty security blanket, steps onto the stage to recite the Christmas story. As he begins reading from Luke 2, he reaches the part where the angel appears to the shepherds and says, *"Fear not."*

At that exact moment, Linus does something he never does—he drops his blanket.

That blanket had always been his source of comfort, his safety net. But as soon as he hears the words, *"Fear not,"* he instinctively lets it go. Why? Because true security isn't found in something we hold onto; it's found in something greater.

That something greater is the hope that God is with us. No matter what we face, we are not alone. Our heavenly Father isn't watching from a distance—He is right there in the middle of it with us. Hope isn't just wishful thinking—it's the anchor that keeps us steady when anxiety tries to pull us under. And when we truly grasp that God is with us, fear loses its grip, and peace takes its place.

Anxiety keeps us clinging to whatever makes us *feel* safe. Maybe it's control, a routine, a relationship, a job, or even avoidance of the things that make us uncomfortable. But those things aren't keeping us safe; they're just security blankets. And just like Linus, we'll only drop them by putting our trust in something greater.

Linus dropped his blanket because, at that moment, he recognized a deeper truth—hope had arrived. And that hope had a name: Jesus. With Him on the scene, fear didn't get the final word anymore.

The same message the angel delivered to the shepherds in Luke 2 is the one Christ delivers to us today: *Fear not. I've got this.*

When we recognize that our security isn't in our circumstances, abilities, or even our sense of control—but in Him—we can finally drop the blanket and walk in real peace.

Hope is among the most powerful weapons in the spiritual battle against anxiety. Hope is "a feeling of expectation and desire for something to happen; a feeling of trust."[17]

That definition highlights an important connection: Hope and trust go hand in hand.

Trust is the choice we make. Hope is the confident feeling that follows.

It works like this:

Anxiety says, *This is never going to get better.*
Hope says, *God is still working.*

Anxiety says, *I'm stuck here forever.*
Hope says, *God makes a way where there is no way.*

Anxiety says, *I'm not strong enough to handle this.*
Hope says, *God's strength is made perfect in my weakness.*

When we choose to trust God despite the chaos around us (and inside us) and continue in that trust no matter how bad things get, hope is the feeling of confidence that settles in our hearts and minds. And sometimes, when we're struggling to see it for ourselves, we need others to remind us that hope is still there.

When I was deep in my struggle with anxiety, feeling completely drained and stuck, Tori became my lifeline. She gave me a spark of hope that lifted my spirit and kept me going when I wanted to quit.

As I mentioned briefly in the introduction, my battle with anxiety wasn't just a one-time event. That first panic attack—unexpected and totally unwelcome—was just the beginning. They kept coming, randomly and relentlessly, with no warning signs.

At the peak of it all, I hit a wall. I had no motivation to do anything: no excitement to watch my kids play sports, no drive to get through my workouts, no interest in my work, and no energy to take my wife out on a date. Everything that used to bring me joy started to feel like a chore. I was unraveling fast, on the edge of a breakdown I never imagined could happen to someone like me.

I never really grasped the weight of depression until I experienced it firsthand. Up until then, I thought anxiety and depression were two separate struggles. But what I discovered is that they often go hand in hand—one feeding off the other, creating a cycle that's hard to escape.

Anxiety whispers, "Something bad is about to happen." Depression responds, "It doesn't matter—nothing's ever going to change." And together, they can lock you into a loop of fear and hopelessness that won't break on its own.

The craziest part? From the outside looking in, I had no reason to feel depressed. I had everything I could ever want—a strong marriage, healthy kids who loved Jesus, thriving businesses, financial freedom, deep friendships, and physical health. So why on God's green earth was I struggling? It made no sense, and that only made it worse.

I was dumbfounded, frustrated, and heartbroken by what was happening inside me.

One morning, after the kids had left for school, I sat in front of our fireplace, feeling completely drained. I had nothing left to give. Then, out of nowhere, Tori walked up behind me and wrapped her arms around me. It felt like a warm blanket for my soul. She leaned in and said, "I was praying for you this morning, and I feel like God wants you to know that this is almost over. It's coming to an end soon. And you're not alone. He's right there with you."

When those words left her mouth, tears started rolling down my cheeks. I wasn't instantly healed. I still had a fight ahead of me. But I felt a weight lift for the first time in a long time. She had given me exactly what I needed to keep going—hope. And sometimes, that's all it takes to keep fighting.

THE VALLEY OF THE SHADOW

King David knew what it meant to hold on to hope in the darkest moments. One of the things I love about the Bible is that God chose to include a man's personal prayer journal in His Word. In the Psalms, we get a raw, unfiltered look at David's heart—a man who battled fear, doubt, and anxiety just like we do (probably even more). In one of his most famous entries, he paints a picture of how terrifying things had become.

"Even though I walk through the valley of the shadow of death ... " (Psalm 23:4a).

It wasn't just death he was facing—it was the *Valley* of the *Shadow* of Death. This wasn't some mountaintop moment where he and God were having a joyful stroll. This was deep in the valley, the kind of place where danger lurks, where every shadow plays tricks on your mind, and where the worst part isn't just the fear of dying, but the fear of dying alone.

He wasn't simply being followed by death itself, but death's shadow. Shadows are always bigger than the real thing. They distort reality, stretching and twisting what's in front of us into something far more terrifying than it actually is. A wolf is scary enough, but its shadow? It looks monstrous. The shadow of death looms large, casting fear and uncertainty over everything in its path.

But here's the thing—shadows can't hurt you. They have no substance, no real power. The Valley of the Shadow of Death wasn't about facing death itself—it was about walking through the fear that death projected. It was the *anticipation* of death.

And that's exactly how anxiety works. It doesn't need real danger to control you; it just needs to cast a big enough shadow to make you believe the worst is coming.

How did David make it through this terrifying valley? The rest of the verse gives us the answer:

"I will fear no evil, for you are with me ..." (Psalm 23:4b).

David factored in the Father. He knew that God was beside him, no matter how dark and dangerous things seemed. And if God was with him, fear had no real power. He didn't have to rely on his strength—he could surrender control, trusting that God would protect him. That was his source of hope and what carried him through the valley.

This verse was written centuries before the disciples' legendary meltdown on the boat when death's shadow seemed to stretch across the stormy sea. Imagine if, instead of panicked screams, Jesus woke up to them declaring, *"Even though we walk through the valley of the shadow of death, we will fear no evil, because your Son is with us!"*

That would have been a next-level display of faith—faith projected into the future instead of fear. Why? Because they would have recognized the most important truth: God was with them. And that truth would have filled them with hope, even in the middle of the storm.

Hudson Taylor, one of the most influential missionaries of all time, perfectly summarized this message:

"All God's giants have been weak men who did great things for God because they reckoned on Him being with them."

When you recognize your hope that God is with you and truly believe that breakthrough is possible because of Him, it changes everything. Fear loses its grip. Anxiety shrinks back into the shadows where it belongs. Your confidence shifts from your strength to His strength, which never fails.

So, the next time fear looms large, remember you are not alone. God is with you, and hope will carry you through.

CHAPTER 8

RECOGNIZE WHAT
YOU'RE FEELING

"Listen to your body's whispers before they become screams!"
–Unknown

～～～

God is always speaking—our job is to make sure we listen. His voice isn't distant or reserved for a select few; it's constant, woven into every moment of our lives. But if we're not tuned in, we'll miss it.

You'll hear His voice in many places when you align your heart to God's frequency. You'll hear Him whispering through Scripture, speaking through the wisdom of a trusted friend, nudging you through a sudden realization, and even confirming things through the circumstances around you. Sometimes, He's loud—like a thunderclap that grabs your attention. Other times, He's subtle—like a gentle breeze reminding you He's near. But make no mistake, God is always speaking.

One of the most powerful—yet often overlooked—ways God gets your attention? Your body. That nagging exhaustion, the tension in your chest, the restlessness you can't shake? Those aren't just random discomforts; they're signals. Your body is the temple of the Holy Spirit, and when something feels off, it's often a divine nudge telling you it's time to pause, reset, or take action.

In this chapter, we will explore two key ways to tune into God's frequency so you'll know exactly how to respond when anxiety creeps in. When you feel that wave of anxiety rising, here's what you do:

- **Listen** to what God is saying.
- **Label** what you're feeling.

Listening and labeling will help you recognize what's happening inside you so you can address it instead of being ruled by it.

Let me show you how this played out in my life.

One of the most interesting books I've written was my fourth, *Bold and Broken*. My brother and I had already tackled the importance of standing strong in your faith with our other books, but we wanted to take it a step further this time. We didn't want to talk about simply *taking* a stand—we wanted to show what happens when you *do*. When you stand for Jesus, you don't just make a statement; you become a bridge—connecting heaven and earth, bringing God's love and truth into the world around you.

Instead of writing *Bold and Broken* the way we had tackled our previous books—where I'd do a massive content dump into a blank document and David would come in for the power edit—we decided to try something different. Our schedules were insane, and we didn't have time to crank out 2,000 words a day on our own. So, we hired an editor, flew him into town for a few days, and dictated the book to him.

The idea was for him to take what we discussed, convert it into a book format, and then send it to us for review and editing. That way, he could handle the heavy lifting of writing while we kept sprinting at a cheetah's pace, building our businesses.

But something about it didn't sit right with me. I felt a knot in my stomach, like I was abandoning something important. It was that same sinking feeling you get when you pat your pockets and realize your phone is missing. Or worse, like driving away from a gas station and suddenly realizing you left one of your kids behind. (Tori: *One of my greatest fears when the kids are with Jason, if I'm honest!*) But every time I looked at my overloaded schedule, I reminded myself this was the right move.

So the editor flew into town and spent a few days with us, during which we verbally laid out the entire book. He recorded everything, assured us he'd have a manuscript ready in six weeks, and then we returned to our busy lives.

But every time I thought about the book, that uneasy feeling crept back into my gut. It wasn't overwhelming, just a nagging little knot that wouldn't go away. I kept brushing it off, reminding myself how packed my schedule was—there was no way I could carve out time to sit and write the book myself. Besides, when I ran it by my closest friends and family, they all agreed it was a smart move.

"You've got too much on your plate," they said. "Let someone else carry the load." Their agreement made it easier to ignore the tension in my spirit.

About a month later, the manuscript arrived. The timing couldn't have been better. We had been hosting our daughter's birthday party in the backyard that day, and after hours of little girls running, screaming, and eating way too much sugar, I slipped onto the back deck, excited for a quiet moment to read through it.

That is, until my internal alarm started blaring so loud I couldn't even focus on another word. Two pages in, and I knew—it was all wrong. The editor had taken what we said and turned it into something completely different. Every sentence felt foreign, and that uneasy feeling in my stomach turned from a little knot to a full-blown wrecking ball.

Then, like a swarm of bees, panic descended. My heart started pounding, my face burned, and a wave of dizziness hit me. The knot in my gut? Now, it felt like a flaming boulder. I slammed my laptop shut, stormed into my room, and started pacing like a man plotting revenge.

And I wasn't just mad at the editor—I was angry at God. *Why would You let this happen?* I thought, as I paced back and forth. *I'm writing this book for You! This is a disaster. There's no way we'll meet the deadline now!*

My dad once told me, "If you love God for what He gives you, you'll hate Him for what He takes from you." And in that moment, it felt like God was taking away the very thing I was trying to do for Him.

Ever been there?

I spent the rest of the day stewing—frustrated at the editor, frustrated at God, and, for good measure, frustrated at David (because why not?). But you know who I *wasn't* mad at? Myself. *What did I do wrong?* As far as I was concerned, I had made the logical decision.

That night, I crawled into bed with the same burning frustration in my gut, and no amount of tossing and turning could ease the tension.

The following day, I woke up early, stepped outside under the stars, and did what had become my routine—talking to God out in nature. The crisp morning air hit my face, the wind rustled through the trees, and the vast sky, sprinkled with stars, stretched above me. At that moment, I felt the unmistakable presence of God.

It wasn't just a feeling but a deep, overwhelming sense of His nearness.

And then, in the stillness, I heard it—not an audible voice, but a quiet stirring in my spirit:

I chose you to write this book. You don't have to do it—it's your choice. But I want you to do it. And if you do, I'll help you.

The words hit me hard. I hadn't heard them the day before, not through all the noise of my frustration and stress. But out there, in the silence, away from the chaos, I could finally listen. And that changed everything.

My immediate reaction was the same as before—*I can't do it! I don't have the time. I* ...

The more I rattled off excuses, the stronger I felt the pull to do it. And the more I resisted, the more that burning sensation in my gut crept back.

But I wanted it gone. Desperately.

And then, something incredible happened—so powerful that I can still picture it vividly.

I stopped pacing. I stopped arguing. I stopped trying to wiggle my way out of it. I dropped to my knees, lifted my hands toward heaven, and surrendered—not because I felt like it, but because I knew it was the right decision. Every part of me wanted to resist, but at that moment, I chose obedience over my emotions.

"Okay, God," I said. "I'll do it. If you want me to write this book myself, I'll do it. Forgive me for running from this responsibility."

In that instant, the weight I had been carrying lifted. The burning in my gut? Gone—like it had evaporated into thin air. A surge of energy and relief rushed through me, unlike anything I had ever experienced.

I felt free—completely and utterly free—like an eagle soaring high above the mountains, unburdened and limitless.

I knew the road ahead wouldn't be easy, but that single moment of surrender gave me the strength I needed to take the first step. I put a simple plan in place and committed to writing a little every day, and the book was finished three months later. And to this day, the introduction—where I shared a portion of this story—remains one of my favorite chapters I've ever written.

The best part of this story isn't that I finished the book. It's that I discovered how God speaks to me through my body. That uneasy feeling? It was His way of nudging me, letting me know I was on the wrong path. That growing knot in my stomach? It was His guidance, urging me toward the direction I was supposed to take.

I needed to listen—to actually pay attention to what my body was trying to tell me. But that wasn't enough. I also needed to label what I was feeling.

All those uncomfortable sensations—the tightness in my chest, the knot in my stomach that felt like it was on fire—that wasn't anxiety. It was *guilt*. And it wasn't until I fully surrendered to God that the Holy Spirit revealed it to me.

And here's the wild part: just like Satan uses fear to hijack your nervous system and launch you into fight-or-flight mode, God can use that very same system to lead you back to Him. That's how brilliant He is! The discomfort I felt wasn't an attack—it was the goodness of God, nudging me to course-correct. But I needed the Spirit's help to recognize that.

I've since learned that conviction and anxiety can feel eerily similar. That's why, back in Chapter Five, we told you that the first step in getting to the root of your anxiety is asking God if there's any sin in your life. Whether the answer is yes or no, starting there clears the table and allows you to focus on what's really going on.

For me, I was ducking my responsibility. But when I got honest with God and repented for running from what I knew I was supposed to do, my guilt lifted and was replaced with gratitude. Suddenly, I had clarity, peace, and the energy to move forward. (We'll talk more about this in Chapter 20.)

Satan doesn't want you to experience conviction. He knows it leads to repentance and freedom. So, instead, he hijacks conviction and calls it anxiety, keeping you stuck in confusion. I could have easily tried to medicate those overwhelming feelings away, but if I had, I wouldn't have addressed the real issue—that I was running from God. In doing so, I forfeited the authority and peace that come with obedience.

I had taken the wrong path, and that burning in my stomach wasn't just random discomfort—it was God's way of pointing me back in the right direction. He wasn't punishing me; He was redirecting me.

This is why listening comes before labeling. If we don't stop and listen, we'll misdiagnose what we're feeling. We'll call it anxiety when it's really conviction. We'll label it as stress when it's actually fear. We'll mistake it for exhaustion when it's avoidance. But when we take the time to listen, God helps us label what's truly going on. And once we name it, we can deal with it.

Remember, an emotion is an impulse to act. You'll move in the wrong direction if you don't label it correctly.

READ THE LABEL

Here are four simple steps to label what you're feeling:

- **Pause and tune in**: When you feel something is a little off, stop for a moment, take a deep breath, and ask yourself: *What exactly am I feeling right now?*

- **Pinpoint where you're feeling it**: Tight chest or racing heart? Maybe it's fear or guilt. Heavy limbs or lack of energy? You could be feeling sadness or exhaustion. Tension in your jaw or fists? Frustration or anger might be at play.

- **Prod for more information**: Ask yourself, *What triggered this feeling? Is there something I need to do or stop doing? Is this reaction proportionate to what's happening?*

- **Pray and ask God for guidance**: You've already been listening to God, but this crucial step shows the importance of continuing the process. Ask God, and keep asking Him, to speak and guide you.

Labeling emotions isn't about getting rid of them—it's about understanding them so they don't control you. When you take the time to name your feelings accurately, you take back the power that anxiety tries to steal from you. And you end up dealing with the actual cause rather than simply addressing the symptom.

If you're looking for a practical tool, try using an Emotion Wheel (sometimes called a Feelings Wheel). You can easily find one online. It's a simple yet effective way to pinpoint what you're feeling. It helps put a name to your emotions, making them easier to process and understand.

When we listen and label, we take back control from the enemy. No more confusion. No more spiraling. Just clarity, direction, and the confidence to take the next step. And when you take that step in obedience, you'll experience what I did—the weight lifts, the fire in your gut fades, and you're finally free to move forward in peace.

And now, here I am writing another book. Go figure.

CHAPTER 9

RECOGNIZE WHAT
YOU'RE THINKING

"The mind is everything. What you think, you become."
–Siddhartha Gautama

Emotions and thoughts are like the classic chicken-and-egg debate: Which comes first? The truth is, they feed off each other. Sometimes, our feelings trigger specific thoughts, and other times, our thoughts stir up particular emotions. Anxiety exploits this cycle, using whichever one it can to pull us deeper into fear, doubt, and confusion.

Have you ever ridden a roller coaster, walked across a high bridge, or done something that triggered a fear response—only for your brain to suddenly start screaming, *This is dangerous! You could die! You might die! You're probably going to die!!* That's a perfect example of emotion leading to thoughts.

On the flip side, have you ever been in the middle of eating a meal when a random thought popped into your head—maybe something stressful or upsetting, or just plain gross—and suddenly, your appetite disappeared? That's thought leading to emotion.

This cycle of thoughts and emotions is what makes anxiety so deceptive—it tricks you into believing that every feeling and every thought is proof that something is wrong. It fuels a constant loop of fear and worry, making it hard to tell what's real and what's not.

The key to breaking free is not just recognizing what you're feeling (as we discussed in the last chapter) but also becoming aware of what you're thinking when anxiety rears its ugly head. And we're not just talking about identifying negative thoughts, although that's important. If you want to overcome anxiety for good, you have to target *ruminating thoughts*—the ones that play on a loop in your mind, keeping you trapped in an endless cycle of fear and doubt.

A ruminating thought is like a broken record in your mind—repeatedly replaying the same fear, mistake, or worry without finding a solution. It's different from problem-solving, which helps you work toward a resolution. Rumination keeps you stuck, convincing you that your worst fears are inevitable.

Instead of a productive thought like, *I made a mistake—how can I fix it?* a ruminating thought sounds more like, *I can't believe I messed up. What if everyone thinks I'm a failure? I'll never recover from this.*

See the difference? One thought moves forward; the other keeps you locked in place.

Rumination is one of anxiety's greatest weapons. The more you dwell on a negative thought, the more power it gains. Left unchecked, ruminating thoughts create an emotional and mental fog that clouds your judgment and drains your energy.

Satan loves to use rumination to keep you stuck. If he can get you replaying past failures or obsessing over what *might* happen, he can keep you from living in the freedom and peace God has for you.

I AM *NOT*

A few days ago, I experienced this firsthand. A guy asked me to look at a commercial building he owns and advise him on what to do with it. I've been investing in real estate for over 20 years—flipping houses, managing rentals, and building a solid portfolio. But do you know the first thought that crossed my mind when I got his text? *I don't know commercial property that well. What if I don't have the right advice? Someone else would probably do a better job.*

Right on cue, I felt that familiar gut reaction—the quick wave of nervousness that whispered, *You don't really know what you're doing. Maybe you should just back out and let someone else handle it.* It was fleeting, but it was real. Had I let my thoughts run unchecked, that tiny feeling could have spiraled into full-blown self-doubt, keeping me from stepping into an opportunity to help someone.

My brother typically handles the commercial side of our real estate business, while I focus on residential. But the truth is, I still know way more about commercial property than 90% of the people out there, including the guy who asked for my advice. Yet, instead of focusing on what I *do* know, my mind immediately fixated on what I *don't* know.

I'm not a commercial real estate expert—true. But does that mean I have nothing to offer? Of course not. I had more knowledge than my friend, and I could absolutely give him solid ideas for his property. But anxiety doesn't let you see reality. It zooms in on what's missing, what's lacking, what *could* go wrong, rather than recognizing what's already there.

Fortunately, I've learned how to shut down thoughts like that before they take root (which you're learning to do in this book). But ten years ago? I probably would have declined the invitation altogether, convinced I'd embarrass myself by standing there like a deer in headlights with nothing to say. Those ruminating thoughts would've kept me stuck—missing an opportunity to help someone who needed my insight.

By the way, I just walked out of that meeting, and you know what? I offered some solid, creative ideas for the building. And he paid for lunch, so it was a double win. (Tori: *Now use those savings and take me to lunch!*)

Negative thoughts will always try to pop into your head—that part's unavoidable. But what *is* avoidable is letting them run wild like kids on a sugar high. And the first step in shutting them down is to shine a light on them—to recognize what you're thinking.

Do you remember what we discussed in Chapter Five—how God's name, Yahweh, means "I AM," declaring Him the ultimate source of power and authority? When we use the powerful name "I AM" and say things like, "I am not smart," "I am not good enough," or "I am not sure I can get through this," we're not just throwing out casual statements— we're reinforcing beliefs that shape our reality. Whether we realize it or not, we're misusing the name of God by assigning power to lies instead of truth.

One of the clearest biblical examples is when God called Moses to lead the Israelites out of Egypt and into the Promised Land. Instead of confidently stepping into his calling, Moses responded just like many of us do when fear and doubt creep in:

"But Moses said to the Lord, 'Oh, my Lord, I am not eloquent, either in the past or since you have spoken to your servant, but I am slow of speech and of tongue'" (Exodus 4:10).

Moses gave power to his doubts by saying "I am" followed by a negative. No wonder God pushed back:

"Then the Lord said to him, 'Who has made man's mouth? Who makes him mute, or deaf, or seeing, or blind? Is it not I, the Lord?'" (Exodus 4:11).

In other words, "Moses, you're focusing on the wrong 'I AM.' It's not about what you lack but who I am!"

When we attach negativity to "I am," we reinforce the very fears and insecurities that hold us back. But here's the good news—you don't have to agree with those thoughts! The next time you catch yourself thinking like Moses, stop and recognize what's happening. Don't give those negative thoughts the power they crave.

Winning the battle against anxiety starts with recognizing the game it plays in your mind. Once you do, you can take control of the narrative and stand with confidence.

IT'S NOT WHAT YOU THINK

One of the ruminating thoughts I found myself stuck in was being anxious about anxiety itself. It was like anxiety had cloned itself— worrying about the possibility of feeling anxious would trigger the very thing I was trying to avoid. I'd be having a great day, feeling totally fine, and then a thought would creep in: *I really hope that wave of anxiety doesn't hit today.* And just like that, I'd start replaying all the awful sensations that come with it—and before I knew it, I was right back in the middle of a full-blown anxiety episode.

That's exactly what happened right before I went on stage to speak at an event in Orlando, Florida. I hadn't had an anxiety attack in months. I was confident, calm, and convinced my worst days were behind me. But just thirty minutes before stepping on stage, those all-too-familiar sensations returned—heart racing, face flushed, palms sweating.

Panic set in: *Oh no, it's happening again! I thought I was past this!* My mind spiraled. I feared I would pass out on stage in front of everyone. I slipped away to the green room, laid down on the floor, and propped my feet on the couch, trying to force blood back to my head. Lying there, fear and sadness collided. I thought, *If this is what happens every time I speak, maybe I shouldn't speak anymore.*

I prayed. I quoted Scripture. I breathed deeply. I tried everything I'd learned. And then, out of nowhere, I remembered something: the vitamin C packet I had dumped into my water earlier. I walked over to the table, picked up the wrapper, and scanned the label. And there it was—in tiny print: "Not recommended for individuals sensitive to caffeine."

It hit me like a lightning bolt—I wasn't having an anxiety attack. I was having a caffeine rush. My body was reacting to something physical, but because my mind interpreted it as anxiety, I immediately spiraled. The moment I realized what was truly happening, the fear began to fade. Just like the false alarm we talked about back in the introduction, this one felt just as real—but it wasn't.

That moment showed me just how damaging ruminating thoughts can be. They have the ability to drag you into panic before anything even goes wrong. When you don't recognize what you're thinking, your mind can become a runaway train—headed straight for fear. But when you *do* stop to recognize the thought, when you catch it in the act and hold it up to the truth, it loses its power.

It was a powerful reminder: when your brain has been conditioned by fear, even a cup of vitamin C can feel like a crisis. But truth is what sets you free. And sometimes, the truth is on the back of the label.

CHAPTER 10

RECOGNIZE WHAT YOU'RE BELIEVING

"Whatever we plant in our subconscious mind and nourish with repetition and emotion will one day become a reality."
–Earl Nightingale

We've discussed the importance of recognizing both the emotions you feel and the thoughts that race through your mind in the battle against anxiety. But what truly fuels both of these—leading either to healing or toward deeper struggle—are the beliefs you hold beneath the surface.

When anxiety strikes—when emotions surge and your thoughts start to spiral—hit pause and ask yourself: *What am I believing right now?* Because belief is what holds the power. It's the foundation that either anchors you in truth or locks you in fear. In that moment, what you choose to believe will determine whether you step into peace or sink further into anxiety.

If your beliefs are anchored in truth, they act as a stabilizing force, helping you navigate emotions in a healthy way and stop anxious thoughts before they spiral. But if your beliefs are rooted in fear, they work like gasoline on a fire—intensifying anxiety and keeping you stuck in its grip.

That's why breaking free from anxiety isn't just about recognizing your thoughts and emotions; it's about identifying the beliefs underneath them. Belief is either the chain that holds you down or the key that sets you free.

Back in Chapter Seven, when I told you how Tori spoke words of hope into me during my most challenging time, my breakthrough didn't come simply because she spoke truth—it came because I *chose to believe* the truth she spoke. Her words were like a life raft tossed into stormy waters, but I had to reach out and grab hold of them. It wasn't her words that gave my emotions power—my *belief* in those words fueled my thoughts.

Tori experienced the same thing in the story she shared in Chapter Six. It wasn't until she truly believed the words she spoke that she was set free from her fear. That belief pushed her toward the goal line instead of dragging her deeper into the pit of anxiety.

And that's the choice you face every time anxiety knocks on the door. Will you believe the lies that keep you stuck (and make it worse)? Or will you choose to believe that what God says is true?

Because what you believe—at the deepest level—will ultimately determine whether you stay trapped in fear or step into the freedom that's already yours.

Now let's get uber-practical. Stay with us on this, because it will feel a little like mental gymnastics. But if you get it, it will help you immensely.

In the last chapter, we mentioned that emotions and thoughts are cyclical. Well, beliefs are as well. Beliefs, emotions, and thoughts all influence each other in a continuous loop. Here's what it looks like in real life.

Your core beliefs—what you hold to be true about God, yourself, others, and the world—act like filters. They shape how you interpret experiences, which in turn determines your thoughts and emotions.

Consider these two examples—one rooted in a lie and the other grounded in truth:

Example 1 (Rooted in a Lie):

- **Belief**: *I'm not good enough.*
- **Thought**: *I'll probably fail this project.*
- **Emotion**: Anxiety, self-doubt, discouragement.

Example 2 (Rooted in Truth):

- **Belief**: *God is in control, and I'm prepared.*
- **Thought**: *This situation is tough, but He will help me.*
- **Emotion**: Peace, confidence, hope.

See how that works? Belief leads to the thought that leads to the emotion.

On the flip side, repeated thoughts and emotions can reinforce or even create new beliefs. If someone repeatedly thinks, "I always mess up," and feels anxious every time they try something new, over time, that thought-emotion pattern can turn into a core belief: "I am a failure."

Here's what it looks like when thoughts take the lead:

Example 1 (Based on a Lie):

- **Thought**: *I can't do this.*
- **Emotion**: Fear and overwhelm.
- **Repeated over time → Belief**: *I'm incapable of handling challenges.*

Example 2 (Based on Truth):

- **Thought**: *God has been faithful before.*
- **Emotion**: Peace and trust.
- **Repeated over time → Belief**: *God will always provide.*

A repeated thought fuels an emotion, which then solidifies into a belief.

Our beliefs shape our thoughts and emotions, but the reverse is also true—our thoughts and emotions can either strengthen or challenge our beliefs. And so, the cycle keeps turning.

What you believe shapes how your mind and body respond. If you believe that the things beyond your control are threats, your thoughts will spiral, your emotions will intensify, and your body will react with stress and anxiety. But if you believe that God is in control and will protect you, your mind will settle, your emotions will stabilize, and your body will follow suit. It might not happen immediately, but it will in time.

YOU'VE GOTTA BELIEVE!

Remember our "not-so-sweet" friend from Chapter Six—the Wicked Witch in Oz? She is the perfect picture of Satan, who does everything he can to rob you of your power. And what was it that led to her ultimate demise?

Water.

And just like the Witch was powerless against a simple splash of water, Satan is powerless against the living water of the Holy Spirit.

But here's what we haven't discussed yet—how do you tap into this living water? Jesus gives the answer:

"Whoever believes in me, as Scripture has said, 'Out of his heart will flow rivers of living water'" (John 7:38).

Whoever *believes in* Jesus gets the living water—they receive the power! Believing in God is the key to overcoming the enemy and the anxiety he uses against us.

But what does it mean to *believe*?

James 2:19 reminds us that "even the demons believe" in God—and shudder. So, belief has to be more than acknowledging that God exists. It's not just head knowledge. It's something deeper, something that changes the way we live.

To believe is to commit. It's to operate out of a deep-seated conviction that God is faithful and He will come through, even when your brain and body are telling you otherwise. It's to move forward *as if* His promises are already fulfilled—because they are.

You probably know this verse by heart:

"For God so loved the world that He gave His one and only Son, that whoever believes in Him shall not perish but have eternal life" (John 3:16).

When I started digging into the original language of the phrase "believe in", I stumbled on a Hebrew theologian who opened my eyes to a powerful truth. In its original meaning, "believe" isn't just about mentally agreeing with a truth—it isn't static. It is a continuous action, something you *do*, not just something you *have*.

And the word "in" in Hebrew means *into*. It's not just about believing *in* God as an idea—it's about believing *into* Him. Think of it like stepping *into* a house or *into* a new position. It's a shift, a movement, a transformation.

Believing in God is an activity that moves us from one place *into* another. It takes us from a place of fear and doubt to a place of peace and power.

As my theologian friend puts it:

"Believing is an act of the will that transports us into a new world where all our living is based on a new relationship. There is no faith without activity, just as there is no life without breathing. If you are 'believing into' God, you will breathe, move, grow, feel, think, and change in this new place. Get into it today!"[18]

Belief isn't passive; it's active. It means recognizing the lie you're believing in the moment of anxiety and choosing to trust God's truth over your feelings. It means stepping *into* faith, not just *agreeing* with it.

This type of belief is portrayed beautifully in the story of Charles Blondin, the famous tightrope walker who traversed across Niagara Falls multiple times. In the 1850s, he became a legend for daring tightrope walks across those raging waters. Time and time again, he crossed without fail—walking backward, blindfolded, even carrying a stove to cook an omelet in the middle of the rope. The crowds loved him, marveling at his skill.

Then, one day, Blondin upped the ante. He asked the crowd, "Who here believes I can cross over Niagara Falls again, but this time pushing a wheelbarrow?"

The crowd shouted, *"We believe, we believe!"* And sure enough, Blondin steered the wheelbarrow successfully across the raging waters and back to the riotous applause of the crowd.

"Who here believes I can cross over Niagara Falls again?" he asked. "But this time with a man in the wheelbarrow?"

The crowd could barely control its enthusiasm. *"We believe! We believe!"* they roared.

Blondin replied, "Ok, then, who will be my first volunteer?"

Silence.[19]

The same people who cheered his skill refused to trust him when it required action. They did not believe themselves *into* the wheelbarrow. Their belief had limits—because real belief requires action.

I repeat—to believe is to commit. It's to operate out of a deep-seated conviction that God is faithful and He will come through, even when your brain and body are telling you otherwise. And this is always a *choice*.

Do you believe that God can pull you out of your anxiety? Do you trust that He can get you across the raging waters of doubt and fear when your emotions are screaming and your thoughts are spiraling?

If you find yourself struggling to believe, you're not alone. In the book of Mark, we see a father wrestling with the same doubt. His son was possessed by a demon, and in desperation, he turned to Jesus for help. Watch how this moment unfolds:

"... 'But if you can do anything, have compassion on us and help us.' And Jesus said to him, 'If you can!' All things are possible for one who believes. Immediately, the father of the child cried out and said, 'I believe; help my unbelief!'" (Mark 9:22-24).

You can do the same—ask God to help you believe. Bring your doubt to Him, and then choose to trust. Align your thoughts and actions with the truth, and your emotions will catch up in time.

So the next time anxiety hits, when your emotions start to spiral and your mind races, pause. Ask yourself: *What am I believing right now?* Because, at the end of the day, belief gives power to your thoughts and emotions.

And when you align your belief with truth, you can be like Harry Colcord, the only person known to have ever trusted Charles Blondin and traversed those raging waters. Some say he got into the wheelbarrow, others say he rode on Blondin's back—but either way, he stepped out in faith and entrusted his life to the tightrope walker. He didn't just stand on the sidelines and say, "I believe you can do it!" He proved his belief by taking the ride.

That's the kind of belief that will carry you over the raging waters of anxiety. The kind that doesn't merely acknowledge that God *can* bring you through it, but steps forward and *lets Him.*

The question is—when He calls you to trust Him, will you stay on the shore, or will you get in the wheelbarrow?

CHAPTER 11

RECOGNIZE THE HABITS YOU'VE FORMED

"More than 40% of the actions people perform each day aren't actual decisions but habits."
–Charles Duhigg

N ow that you've taken the time to recognize what you're feeling, thinking, and believing, it's time to take an honest look at the habits you've formed as a result. Because here's the truth: anxiety isn't just a feeling you wrestle with—it's a rhythm you can fall into. Over time, anxious thoughts and reactions can hardwire themselves into your daily routines, shaping how you move through life without you even realizing it.

A habit is "a settled or regular tendency or practice; an automatic reaction to a specific situation."[20] In other words, it's something you do without even thinking about it.

You don't wake up in the morning and debate whether you should brush your teeth—you just do it. You don't have to remind yourself to check your phone when bored—you instinctively reach for it. That's the power of a habit. It's ingrained in your brain, shaping your actions without requiring conscious effort.

This happens because our brains, while acting as the command center of our lives, are constantly looking for ways to work more efficiently and conserve energy. They do this by turning repeated actions into habits so they don't have to process them from scratch every time. Habits serve as mental shortcuts, freeing up brainpower by automating routine tasks and allowing us to focus on more complex decisions.

Research shows that stress increases with the number of decisions we make daily.[21] The more choices we face, the more mentally drained we become. Habits help counteract this by reducing decision fatigue. They allow us to operate on autopilot for everyday actions, freeing up mental energy for what truly matters.

Our brains don't only create shortcuts to save energy—they also do it to avoid discomfort. Habits are the brain's way of handling anything uneasy or uncertain. They're not just about making life more convenient; they're survival mechanisms designed to help us navigate challenges with as little resistance as possible.

Let's say you hit a wall on a work project. You're tired and stressed, and you just need a break. Next thing you know, you're in the kitchen smashing that box of thin mint Girl Scout cookies your daughter put in the fridge. Before you know it, you're no longer thinking about the problem, which results in decreased frustration and stress. Your brain recognizes that this little process worked and subconsciously jots a mental note—*eating sugar delivers a reward in the form of stress reduction*—and will return to it again and again.

Just like that, a habit is born.

Habits allow us to move through life without overthinking every little thing—like how to tie our shoes, drive a car, or make our coffee. But here's the catch: the brain doesn't distinguish between helpful and harmful habits. It simply automates whatever we repeatedly do. Only our conscious mind can recognize the difference.

Smashing Girl Scout cookies when frustrated might feel good at the moment and diminish your stress, but your body will pay for it. Do that long enough, and the scale in your bathroom might respond, "To Be Continued." Your body suffered because your brain wanted a break.

Your brain is the VIP concierge of your life—always trying to make things easier and more comfortable for you. Think of it like Mr. Hector, the maitre d' at the Plaza Hotel in *Home Alone 2*. Remember that guy? His sole mission was to cater to young Kevin McCallister's every whim. And before you know it, 10-year-old Kevin is sprawled out in a penthouse suite, surrounded by candy, living his best life while inhaling a giant bowl of ice cream—not two scoops, but three—because, let's be honest, *he's not driving!*

The moment your brain senses discomfort, it's pushing you toward the easy, feel-good option—hit the bar, not the gym. Grab the Cheetos, not the kale salad. The good news? You can train it to pick the better option. We'll get to that in Step Three.

Now, let's apply habits to anxiety. Anxiety doesn't just affect how you feel—it trains your brain, shaping the way you react to discomfort, fear, and uncertainty. Over time, repeated anxious thoughts and feelings create habits to avoid perceived threats or provide quick relief. The problem? These habits might feel helpful at the moment, but they actually reinforce the anxiety, keeping you stuck in the same exhausting cycle.

Maybe you've habitually avoided certain situations just because they make you uncomfortable. Or perhaps the moment anxiety creeps in, you instinctively check out, distract yourself, or numb the feeling. Or maybe you've developed a habit of overthinking, constantly running through worst-case scenarios before you even realize what you're doing. Sound familiar? That's anxiety turning into a habit.

Take a moment to ask yourself: *What habits do I fall into when I feel uncomfortable?* Seriously, stop and think about it for a second.

Here's the thing—bad habits don't vanish into thin air. You can't wake up one day and simply decide to stop an ingrained response. But here's the good news: just like your brain, habits can be rewired.

To break anxiety-driven habits, you first have to recognize them. What behaviors have you adopted as a way to cope with fear? What thought patterns automatically start looping in your mind when anxiety creeps in?

Any mental, emotional, or physical habit can keep you stuck or set you free. Once you become aware of your patterns, you gain the power to change them for the better.

To help you do this, let's break down how habits work and the process for rewiring them.

In *The Power of Habit*, Charles Duhigg identifies three key components that make up every habit:

- **Cue** – The trigger that signals your brain to slip into autopilot and engage in a habit.
- **Routine** – The habit itself (whether mental, emotional, or physical).
- **Reward** – The perceived "positive" outcome that reinforces the habit.

Understanding this cycle is the key to breaking old habits and building healthier ones. Think of this as your personal "CRR code"—your unique, automatic way of responding to triggers. Every habit you've developed follows this same Cue-Routine-Reward pattern, whether you realize it or not.

Let's go back to our earlier work project example.

- **Cue:** You hit a wall in your project and feel frustrated and stressed.
- **Routine:** You head to the kitchen and start crushing some snacks.
- **Reward:** The frustration fades (at least temporarily), and the sugar gives you a dopamine boost.

According to Duhigg, changing a habit works best when you keep the same cue and reward but swap out the routine—this is the Golden Rule of habit change. Your brain craves familiarity, so instead of trying to eliminate a habit outright, you replace the existing routine with a new, healthier one while keeping the structure intact.[22]

This trick worked like magic for me, because I had a serious ice cream problem when my kids were little. As any parent will tell you, those early years are pure chaos. By the time we survived the bedtime battle and those little balls of energy were finally asleep, I'd gravitate toward the fridge like it was my life's mission. Right on cue, I'd hear it calling me—like a damsel in distress—and without a second thought, I'd answer. The next thing I knew, half a container of chocolate chip was gone.

The ever-expanding tire around my waist finally convinced me that something had to change. So, I swapped my ice cream routine for a dark chocolate routine. Every night after putting the kids to bed, my cravings kicked in (cue). But instead of heading to the freezer, I'd open the cabinet and grab a block of 70% dark chocolate (routine). At first, it was rough—I mean, let's not pretend dark chocolate is ice cream—but I stuck with it. Over time, my cravings shifted, and eventually, I wanted the dark stuff more than ice cream (reward).

Now? I couldn't care less about ice cream—unless it's homemade chocolate chip from Kilwins. But that's a different story.

The key? Small wins. Just focus on one habit today. Swap out the routine, stick with it, and don't quit. It will get easier and easier until it becomes second nature.

The bottom line is that your brain is wired for efficiency. It craves less effort, less struggle, and less discomfort. It doesn't want to push through the hard stuff; it wants the easiest escape route. If left unchecked, it will run from pain and discomfort every single time.

But when you start recognizing the habits you've built to avoid the discomfort of anxiety, you take a decisive step toward breaking free from them—for good. And in the process, you'll discover a powerful truth, one that's plastered on the walls of CrossFit gyms everywhere:

"More is accomplished in the pain cave than in the comfort zone!"

RECOGNIZE WHAT'S HAPPENING

"Nothing diminishes anxiety faster than action."
–Walter Anderson

The first step to overcoming anxiety and taking back control of your life is **recognition**—learning to spot what's really happening in the moment and identifying the true *enemy* behind it. Satan is the one pulling the strings, and until you recognize the signs of his influence, you'll stay stuck in the mental traps he sets. Awareness is the starting point of freedom.

Once you expose the enemy's schemes, the next step is to shift your focus to the *hope* you have in Christ. As a follower of Jesus, you don't fight *for* victory—you fight *from* it. God is with you and will carry you through, no matter what.

From there, you must begin paying attention to four key areas of your life—each one constantly speaking, if you're willing to listen:

- What you're *feeling* – The emotional and physical responses triggered by anxiety.

- What you're *thinking* – The thought patterns that either fuel fear or build faith.

- What you're *believing* – The truths (or lies) we hold onto.

- What *habits* you've developed – The routines that reinforce our mental, emotional, and spiritual health.

When anxiety creeps in, the enemy always leaves clues that he's behind it. And if we start paying attention to these four key areas, we'll be able to spot him instantly and shut him down before he takes control.

So that's it for Step One - RECOGNIZE. This step is about awareness; the next two steps are about action.

Are you ready to take them?

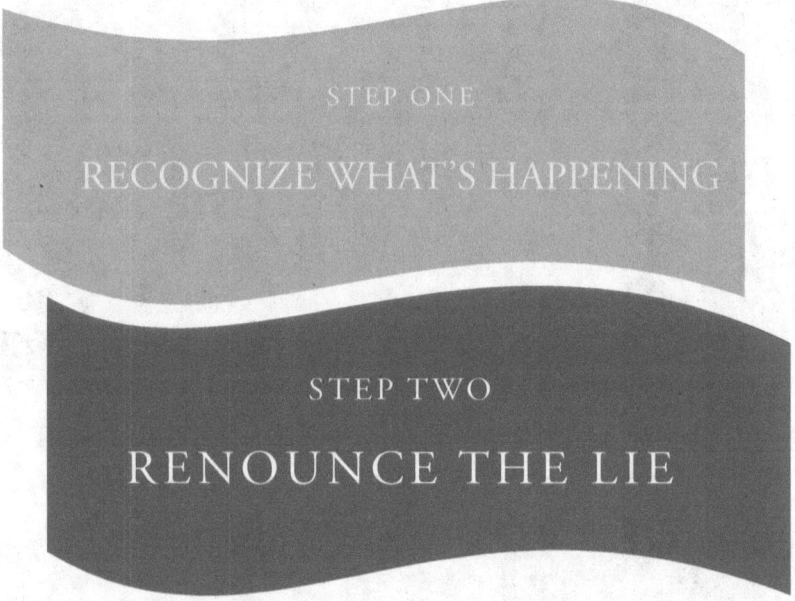

STEP ONE

RECOGNIZE WHAT'S HAPPENING

STEP TWO

RENOUNCE THE LIE

CHAPTER 12

REFUSE TO BELIEVE YOU'RE UNSAFE

"P.S. You're not going to die ... It feels like you are.
It feels like a lion is chasing you.
It feels like a bear has spotted you.
But it's just the anxiety. You're safe."
–Glennon Doyle

Behind every anxious thought is a deception designed to shake our faith. And the most effective lies are the ones that are *almost* true.

Satan knows how to twist reality just enough to make us take the bait, filling our minds with accusations and worst-case scenarios. But here's the key: an accusation only has power if we *agree* with it.

To renounce something means to formally reject it—to abandon it entirely and refuse to let it have any power over you. And if you want to break free from anxiety, the first lie you need to renounce is the one that keeps it alive: the lie that you're unsafe.

If you've ever taught a teenager how to drive, you know exactly how powerful that lie can feel.

We've trained three teenage drivers and are about to start our fourth. And let us tell you—of all the challenges that come with parenting, teaching a teenager to drive ranks right up there with potty training and assembling Christmas gifts with a thousand tiny pieces. It's not just about explaining the rules of the road or dealing with their "I know, I know" attitude. It's because we value our own lives and strongly desire to keep all our limbs intact.

There's something about sitting in the passenger seat with a nervous, heavy-footed teenager behind the wheel that makes you rethink your life. We've feared for *their* safety for years, but the moment they slide into the driver's seat, that fear shifts fast. Suddenly, it's *our* lives flashing before our eyes.

Watching them attempt a left turn at a busy intersection is a full-blown survival exercise—clutching the door handle, stomping on an invisible brake pedal, and whispering desperate prayers we haven't uttered since childhood. Nothing strengthens your faith quite like entrusting your well-being to someone who still forgets to put the milk back in the fridge.

Why do we feel this way? Because deep down, we're wired for safety. We don't want to get hurt, and in that moment, our sense of safety feels anything but certain.

Whether it's a car accident, a fall, or some completely irrational but very real fear, we're wired to avoid danger. It's human nature. But anxiety takes that instinct and cranks it up, making us believe we're unsafe even when there's no real threat.

The problem is that the more we live in fear of getting hurt, the more we focus on how unsafe we are, and the more we'll live in a state of fear rather than freedom. Instead of assessing risk rationally, we start seeing threats where there are none, avoiding perfectly safe situations, and making decisions based on what-ifs rather than reality. Eventually, fear doesn't just protect us from danger—it traps us, limiting what we do, where we go, and who we become.

Remember how we talked in the introduction about God wiring us with an internal alarm system to alert us to danger? That fear response is a gift—it keeps us from walking into traffic or touching a hot stove. But Satan knows how powerful this system is, and that's exactly why he hijacks it. Instead of allowing fear to protect us from real danger, he twists it—convincing us that things that are actually safe are dangerous. And just like that, we start avoiding what God wants us to do and we become paralyzed instead of growing in faith and confidence.

Is it true that we are unsafe in a car with a teenage driver? Yes and no. When I slide into the passenger seat and my 15-year-old daughter grips the wheel like a lifeline, my Level Two Alert System should activate. (Remember that from Chapter Four?) My senses should be heightened, I should scan for potential hazards, and I should be more aware of my surroundings than if I were safely parked on my couch, watching TV next to said teenager.

But if I'm not careful, my brain will go full NASCAR-wreck highlight reel. Within seconds, I'll start convincing myself that the first intersection we approach is where it all ends—the obituary will read, "Father of four dies in a tragic left-turn hesitation incident."

So what do I do? I refuse to let her drive. Ever.

Fast forward a few years, and now she's 22 years old, a college senior, and still hitching rides like a lost freshman because she's the only one in her friend group who never got a license.

Moral of the story? Fear will keep you "safe," alright—safe in your comfort zone, where nothing ever happens, nothing ever changes, and both you and the people you love stay stuck, never becoming who God created you to be.

Thankfully, for us and our daughter, that story was purely hypothetical. But it makes a powerful point: of all the lies anxiety throws your way, the idea that you're unsafe is one of the most crippling.

If Satan can convince you that danger is always right around the corner, he doesn't have to block your path—he just has to make you too scared to walk it. Fear will do the rest.

He'll target your beliefs, making you question whether God is truly your protector. He'll hijack your emotions, flooding you with fear until it feels impossible to move forward. He'll seize control of your thoughts, filling your mind with worst-case scenarios that make even the smallest risks feel life-threatening. Finally, he'll rewire your habits, training you to avoid anything that feels uncertain, uncomfortable, or unknown—all in the name of "staying safe."

Before you know it, you're stuck—not because danger is truly present, but because you've shaped your life around avoiding an alarm designed to warn, not confine.

Why does this happen? Because your #1 core human need is security—the assurance that you are safe. Your brain constantly scans your environment, asking, *Am I safe here? Are these people safe? Is this situation safe?* If the answer is yes, you move forward without hesitation. But if the answer is no, everything stops.

Think about checking into a hotel room only to realize the door won't lock. How well are you going to sleep? You won't! No matter how exhausted you are, your brain and body won't let you relax until you feel secure. Instead of peacefully drifting off, you'll spend the night in a half-sleep daze, jolting awake at every sound, double-checking the makeshift barricade you built from a desk chair and your suitcase. Because when security is missing, rest is too.

God wired us with the need for security because He wants us to find our security in Him.

The more unsafe we feel, the more we are meant to look to Him as our refuge. This need is built into us from birth—just like a baby instinctively reaches for a parent when they feel scared, we are designed to reach for our Heavenly Father in moments of uncertainty.

David understood this better than anyone. Throughout the book of Psalms, we see him—a man constantly pursued and threatened by enemies inside and out—declare a powerful truth:

"God is our refuge and strength, a very present help in trouble" (Psalm 46:1).

Refuge means "a condition of being safe or sheltered from pursuit, danger, or trouble."[23] David wasn't naïve—he knew danger was real. He took precautions and made plans. But he also knew that at some point, no amount of preparation, strategy, or human effort could guarantee his safety—only God could do that.

So, instead of letting his mind spiral into fear and insecurity, David anchored himself in truth. He intentionally chose to trust God as his refuge. And that's the choice we have to make, too.

Because here's the reality: you will feel unsafe sometimes. Anxiety will tell you that you're in danger when you're not. Fear will try to convince you that safety is found in avoiding, controlling, or running away. But you have to refuse to believe the lie that you are unprotected.

Your security does not come from your circumstances. It comes from God alone. And when you place your trust in Him—not in your ability to control outcomes—you'll finally be able to silence anxiety and walk in peace.

And let's be honest—God is a much better driving instructor than we are. No panic stomping on imaginary brakes, no gripping the door handle like a lifeline, and no screaming "BRAKE! BRAKE! BRAKE!" at the last second.

God's got this—so go ahead and unclench your jaw.

CHAPTER 13

REFUSE TO ASSUME CONTROL

*"Suffering arises from trying to control
the uncontrollable, or from neglecting
what is within our power."*
—Epictetus

~

Remember when Carrie Underwood came out with "Jesus Take the Wheel"? That song shot to #1 faster than a grandma spotting a clearance rack. It was everywhere—playing in grocery stores, gas stations, dentist offices. You couldn't go anywhere for more than ten minutes without hearing someone belt out, "Jesus, take the wheeeeeel!"

And then, of course, Tim Hawkins gave us the true masterpiece—his spoof "Cletus Take the Reel." I have to admit that one spoke to me. But I digress.

So why did "Jesus Take the Wheel" resonate with so many people? Because it puts words to something we all struggle with—letting go of control. Deep down, we know we're not meant to run the show, yet we cling to the illusion that if we just grip the wheel hard enough, plan well enough, and stress about every possible outcome, we can somehow steer life exactly where we want it to go.

But control is a sneaky little liar. It tricks us into believing we're safe if we hold on tight. In reality, the tighter we grip, the more anxious we become. We white-knuckle the steering wheel of life, convinced that if we loosen our grip even a little, everything will spin out of control.

Anxiety feeds off this need for control. It whispers, "If you don't manage every detail, something will go wrong." It convinces us that we have to micromanage every outcome, predict every scenario, and stay two steps ahead.

Refusing to assume control means shifting from "I have to figure everything out" to "God already has this figured out." We finally make space for real peace when we stop gripping the wheel like our lives depend on it.

NO LIMBS, NO PROBLEM

The best example I can share of someone who has every reason to feel out of control—but refuses to live in fear—is my good friend, Nick Vujicic. Here's a man with no arms and legs, someone the world might assume is entirely at the mercy of his circumstances. And yet, Nick is among the most joyful, fearless, and faith-filled people I've ever known.

I saw this firsthand when we took a beach vacation with Nick and his family in the Florida Keys. A group of us guys took off on a boat, cruising about 45 minutes from the house, with Nick and his two sons along for the ride. And then, out of nowhere, the sky turned on us. Massive storm clouds rolled in fast, and within minutes, we were clearly in trouble.

Our boat captain said there was no way we'd make it back before the storm hit. So he told us we'd have to find a way to get out and hitch a car ride back to the house.

The only problem? We couldn't get the boat close enough to the beach, and no docks were in sight. That meant we had only one option—jump into four feet of water and trek to shore, about 75 yards away.

My brother was the first to take the plunge. I passed Nick to him and jumped in after, beginning the long, grueling trek to shore. David took the lead, and I followed closely behind.

Let me tell you—this was no casual stroll. Every step was a battle, our feet sinking deep into the thick mud like quicksand. The moment we'd manage to yank one foot free, a wave would hit, knocking us off balance and shoving us two steps back. It was part rescue mission, part full-body workout.

I yelled at David, "Let me take Nick so you can take a break!"

He shook his head and shouted, "I CAN'T STOP—MOMENTUM!" He was afraid the waves would've knocked him over if he stopped.

We had about 30 yards to go before reaching the beach, and I couldn't shake the growing fear that David might drop Nick. We had been trekking for about three minutes, and I could see David's body visibly shaking as he struggled to hold on. To make matters worse, I was just far enough behind them that if he dropped him, I wasn't sure I'd reach him before he started drifting out to sea.

It was a crazy, surreal moment—one of those times where you're half-panicked, half-thinking, *Is this real life?*

But the most incredible part? Nick's face. You'd think he'd be panicked, bracing for the worst, maybe even screaming, "SAVE ME, JESUS!" But nope. The guy was as calm as could be. Instead of freaking out, he was encouraging David the whole way.

"You got this, bro. You can do it."

Meanwhile, David was basically auditioning for an episode of *Survivor*, his legs shaking with every step. When we were about five feet from shore, Nick joked, "You're almost there ... don't drop me now!"

We made it. When we hit solid ground, I yanked Nick out of David's arms, and David collapsed like he had just completed an Ironman. I looked at him and said, "You'll never get another compliment from me, but that was impressive."

But the most impressive thing wasn't David's heroic feat—it was Nick's unshakeable calm. He wasn't spiraling into anxiety, worrying about what he couldn't do, or stressing over what was out of his control. Instead, he did what he's learned to do his whole life—surrender his limitations to God, choosing trust over fear.

Later, Nick admitted he was a little nervous (who wouldn't be?). But he didn't panic. He said he knew David had the strength to make it—he just needed encouragement to keep going. And that's what made it so powerful.

Peace doesn't come from being in control. It comes from knowing who is in control. And in that moment, God had David on the job.

At the end of the day, Nick's trust isn't in a person—it's in God. And his life completely debunks the myth that control is what keeps us safe. If that were true, he'd be the most anxious person on the planet. Instead, he's the opposite—fully surrendered, fully trusting, and entirely at peace.

Nick's story is living proof that real freedom comes when we stop gripping for control and start placing our faith in God. The moment we do, anxiety loses its power, fear fades, and we step into the peace we were meant to have all along.

So what can you do when you feel the urge to grab control and take the wheel from Jesus instead of letting Him stay in the driver's seat? Saying, "Just trust God, and it'll all work out," sounds nice, but is that all we're supposed to do?

While trusting God is the right mindset, there's still a part you have to play.

Here's your role:

Take responsibility for what you can and should control—then leave the rest to God.

STACKING PENNIES

I saw this firsthand through another good buddy, Corey LaJoie, a nine-year NASCAR veteran. We met up one day to catch up on life, and as we talked, he shared something that would have rattled just about anyone.

A few days before our meeting, he had the lead in the Daytona 500 with only three laps to go. And if you know racing, the Daytona 500 is the Super Bowl of NASCAR. Winning that race is a career-defining moment—a dream every driver chases.

But then, everything fell apart. He got tangled up in a crash, and not only did he lose the race—he never even made it to the finish line.

Yet, as he told me the story, he was all smiles and full of joy—no bitterness, no frustration, just peace. I asked him, "How are you handling this so well?"

Without missing a beat, he shrugged and said, "It's the joy of the Lord, man. I mean, I really wanted to win, and yeah, I'm bummed it didn't happen—but I know God's got it all under control."

He went on to tell me that a few years ago, this kind of loss would have wrecked him. Back then, anxiety had a grip on him, and when things didn't go his way, it led to temper flare-ups and emotional outbursts that completely threw him off course.

On top of that, he constantly battled the feeling of failure because his team didn't have the same budget as the bigger ones. Race after race, he found himself finishing in the lower half of the pack, and it ate away at him. No matter how hard he worked, he felt like he was always coming up short.

He felt defeated and exhausted and even considered quitting racing. But then, a fellow driver suggested he meet with a sports psychologist, and that conversation taught him the greatest lesson of his racing career.

She pointed out that in every race, countless factors are entirely out of his control—engine issues, parts failures, pit crew mistakes, or even the fact that his team didn't have the massive budgets of the top-tier teams. No amount of stress or frustration could change those things.

And yet, the more he focused on what he couldn't control—measuring his success by where he finished compared to others—the more frustrated, anxious, and angry he became.

But if he flipped his focus—stopping the obsession over what he couldn't control and instead locking in on what he could—he'd start to reclaim his joy, motivation, and peace. The key wasn't chasing wins but learning to celebrate the small victories that most people overlook or never bother to notice.

Together, they made a list of controllable wins—simple, intentional actions he could take regardless of where he finished in a race. Things like:

- Smile when walking into the garage, no matter how the last race went.
- Never hit the wall on my own—stay focused and steady.
- Optimize pit road speed within 0.3 mph of the limit.
- No cussing over the radio, no matter how frustrating things get.

They called this practice "stacking pennies" because every penny bears the words "In God We Trust." The idea was simple—focus on what you can control and trust God with the rest. It served as a constant reminder to prioritize small, consistent wins rather than getting lost in the uncontrollable chaos of racing.

After each race, Corey would tally up how many "pennies" he collected—not based on his finishing position, but on the things he could control. And no matter the race's outcome, he and his therapist would celebrate each small win.

Slowly but surely, the stack of pennies grew. His mindset shifted, and his joy returned. The frustration that once drained him was replaced with a sense of purpose and peace. Racing was no longer about controlling the uncontrollable; it was about doing his part, trusting God, and letting go of the rest.

And the car he raced in Daytona? It carried the image of a penny, with the words "In God We Trust" just behind the number decal on his door. A testimony of what happens when we stop white-knuckling life, stop chasing control, and start trusting the One who already has it all handled.

Because here's the truth—control was never yours to hold. Anxiety thrives on the illusion that you have to manage every outcome, predict every possibility, and never let your guard down. But peace comes when you refuse to assume control and place your trust where it belongs—in God.

So stack your pennies. Do what you can, and surrender the rest. Ultimately, true freedom isn't found in having control—it's found in knowing who is in control.

CHAPTER 14

REFUSE TO IDENTIFY WITH YOUR ANXIETY

"Your true identity is who God says you are.
You will never discover who you are
by looking inside yourself..."
–David Powlison

Moment of honesty here—all four of our kids were the *climbing-the-walls, human tornado* type. The kind of kids whose naps lasted a whopping 20 minutes and somehow functioned on six hours of sleep a night. (Slight exaggeration ... but only slight.)

There were times we'd take them to the park, and they'd go so wild that Tori would give me *the look* and whisper, "Go get your kids, and let's get out of here!"

Because let's be real—when your kid is terrorizing the playground and causing every other parent to regret the day they discovered that park, you're not exactly eager to take credit.

So why do we do that with anxiety, claiming it as our own?

When we say things like, "I am anxious," or "I have an anxiety disorder," or "My anxiety is acting up," we're claiming ownership of the very thing that's wreaking havoc in our lives—as if anxiety belongs to us, as if it's part of who we are.

Here's the truth: God didn't make you that way.

Go back and read the quote at the top of the chapter. God is the one who defines you. And you are not your struggle. (While we're at it, you're also not your sin—but that's a whole different book.)

The real question is, who does God say you are? Because when you start identifying with who you are in Christ and stop identifying with your anxiety, you can break free from it.

That question reminds me of another song that shot to the top of the global charts faster than our dog, Rocky, shoots into the kitchen when he hears the fridge door opening. (Tori: *Jason won't stop sharing his food with the dog, despite my efforts.*)

I'm talking about "You Say" by Lauren Daigle. You couldn't walk into a mall, step into a coffee shop, or even watch a faith-based movie without hearing, "You say I am loved when I can't feel a thing ..." And for good reason, because it speaks to the core of our identity.

Instead of believing who God says we are, we label ourselves based on our struggles, our emotions, or whatever anxiety is yelling at us at the moment. But feelings don't define you. Anxiety doesn't define you. God does.

The fact that you're *struggling* proves that your anxiety doesn't define you. Why?

Because your identity is determined by what—or to whom—you surrender.

Let me say that again so it sinks in:

Your identity is determined by what—or to whom—you surrender.

If you raise the white flag and stop fighting, you don't just struggle with anxiety—you *become* anxious. If you give in to fear, it takes over. The moment you stop resisting the lie, it becomes your truth.

But here's the good news: You don't have to surrender to your struggle. You can surrender to God instead—and in doing so, step into the identity He has already declared over you. The fight isn't over unless you decide it is.

FULL SURRENDER

The Apostle Paul lays out this principle in his letter to the Corinthians, helping them see their lives through a new lens based on who Jesus is and who they become when they surrender to Him.

These believers struggled with the same things we wrestle with today— past mistakes, destructive habits, and identities shaped by their failures. So Paul gets straight to the point, listing out a laundry list of behaviors they used to engage in before knowing Jesus—things no one would be proud of. You can read 1 Corinthians 6:9-10 to see the list.

But then Paul flips the script:

"And that is what some of you were ... " (1 Corinthians 6:11a).

Before they knew Jesus, their identity was wrapped up in their actions. They "were" those things because they had surrendered to them.

But Paul doesn't leave them there. He reminds them that everything changed the moment they surrendered to Christ:

"... But you were washed, you were sanctified, you were justified in the name of the Lord Jesus Christ and by the Spirit of our God" (1 Corinthians 6:11b).

In other words, you are no longer defined by what you do. Your past no longer owns you, and your struggle is no longer your identity. When you surrendered to Jesus, you became brand new.

Paul understood something powerful about identity:

How you see yourself determines how you behave yourself.

If you *believe* you are your struggle, you will live like it. But if you *believe* you are who God says you are, you will start walking in that truth.

How are believers supposed to see themselves? What is our new identity? Paul answers that question in his letter to the Romans:

"For those who are led by the Spirit of God are the children of God" (*Romans 8:15*).

We are God's kids! Our identity isn't found in our sin, struggle, or past mistakes—it is found in our Father.

Take a moment and let that sink in.

I know I picked on my kids earlier, but let me make this clear—there is absolutely nothing I wouldn't do for them. I don't care how squirrelly, chaotic, or off-the-walls they've been—they are my kids. And because they're mine, whatever power and resources I have are available to them.

And guess what? God says the same about you!

When you surrender to God, He adopts you as His own. You become His kid. You're no longer just someone struggling through life, barely holding it together. You are a child of the all-powerful, sovereign ruler of the universe—the great "I AM." His name defines identity itself.

This is why we must never use God's name to create false identities. When we say things like "I am anxious" or "I am a failure," we speak falsehood over the identity He gave us, giving those lies power. You might *feel* anxious or like a failure, but that's not who you are.

Because here's the truth: *What you speak, you strengthen.*

You are not ill. You are not sick. You may be struggling right now, but you are not your struggle. Why? Because you're God's kid. Your identity has shifted—you are no longer a slave to fear, anxiety, or anything else that once ruled over you. It may have been your master before, but not anymore.

And here's the best part—since you're God's child, His power flows through you!

"And if the Spirit of him who raised Jesus from the dead is living in you, he who raised Christ from the dead will also give life to your mortal bodies because of his Spirit who lives in you" (Romans 8:11).

In other words, everything that belongs to God is available to you!

Think about that. The same powerful Spirit that raised Jesus from the dead lives in you. If He has resurrection power, how much more can He crush anxiety, defeat overwhelm, and conquer the fears that freak you out?

You are not powerless. You are not stuck. You are not your struggle.

Therapy culture often keeps people trapped in an endless cycle of self-exploration, constantly searching *within* for answers. And while self-awareness is valuable, you will never fully discover who you are if that's all you do.

True identity isn't found by looking inward but by looking upward. When you shift your focus to God, you'll finally see who you are, who He created you to be, and the power He's put inside you.

Here's the key—*once you know who you are, don't speak who you're not!*

Words carry weight. They shape your identity. If you speak fear, you strengthen fear. If you speak truth, you strengthen truth.

What you say either builds you up or tears you down. If you constantly repeat, "I'm anxious," "I'm a failure," or "I'll never be enough," those words start to define you. Over time, your brain stops questioning them and simply accepts them as truth.

So make a choice—speak what God says about you. Because in the end, His words are the only ones that actually define you. (We'll show you in Step Three how to practically do this through declarations.)

BREAKING FREE

This hit home with me in a very real way at the height of my struggle with anxiety. At that point, I felt like I was grasping for anything just to stay afloat. I prayed, read books, watched videos, sought counsel—anything that might give me answers.

During that time, I stumbled across the testimony of a guy who had been completely wrecked by anxiety. It had taken everything from him—he couldn't get out of bed, lost his job, and watched his relationships fall apart. His health spiraled as he felt like a prisoner in his own mind.

Anxiety had taken complete control over his life. But then, one morning, he had a moment of crystal-clear realization—as if God Himself was shaking him awake.

He suddenly saw what had been keeping him trapped all along: he had been identifying with his struggle. The very thing he hated—that crushing anxiety—was what he had claimed as his own.

Right then and there, he made a bold decision—he would no longer identify with anxiety and call it "his." He would no longer accept the lie that he was broken or ill. He would stop saying "my anxiety" as if it belonged to him.

Instead of surrendering to the struggle, he started declaring who he was—the strength he had, the victory that was already his. And that was the moment everything changed. That was the moment he broke free.

I don't know if that guy was a believer, but he tapped into a powerful truth—you can break free from anxiety when you refuse to identify with it.

As a believer, your identity isn't defined by fear or failure—it's defined by who God says you are. When you stop identifying with your anxiety, you can break free from it.

Here's the truth: Your feelings don't define you. Anxiety doesn't define you. God does. And He calls you His kid. More than that, you've got His power flowing through your veins.

So don't wave the white flag and surrender to your struggle. Instead, surrender to God. Tap into the power that already belongs to you as His son or daughter.

And one day, your story—the one you're living right now—will be the very thing that helps someone else break free.

In the meantime, crank up "You Say" by Lauren Daigle and let it wash over you. And when you find yourself singing along like you're part of the band, you might as well start believing the lyrics.

CHAPTER 15

REFUSE TO BE DOUBLE-MINDED

*"All the world over, it is true that a
double-minded man is unstable in all his ways,
like a wave... tossed hither and thither
with every eddy of its tide."*
–William Morley Punshon

My dad used to tell my brother and me, "Boys! Don't ever straddle the fence. If you do, you'll tear the seat of your pants." At twelve years old, that mental image alone made us wince. But over time, we understood what he meant—go all in when you make a decision. Otherwise, you'll hurt yourself.

Straddling the fence and being double-minded are basically the same thing. One foot in, one foot out. One foot planted in faith, the other in fear. One moment, you're declaring God's promises with confidence, and the next, you're Googling worst-case scenarios like you're preparing for certain death.

When we're torn between trusting God and trying to control everything ourselves, we become mentally and emotionally unstable—constantly second-guessing, overthinking, and running in circles. Anxiety thrives in that space. And it's exhausting.

We saw this firsthand with a couple we coached a few years ago. They were dealing with some ongoing struggles, most of them rooted in the husband's battle with anxiety—specifically around work and money.

Despite being incredibly successful in business, he was never satisfied with his situation. No matter how much he earned, he constantly worried about money, convinced there was never enough. The irony? There was plenty. But in his mind, scarcity was always lurking around the corner, keeping him in constant fear.

For about three months, we worked with them, trying everything we could think of—but no matter what we did, nothing seemed to stick. Every time he made progress, he'd fall right back to the same anxious patterns. He kept hitting Level Three when he should have been hovering at Level One.

It was hard to watch. But over time, we started noticing that he was consistently distracted, as if he was simultaneously being pulled in a dozen directions.

It showed up in his work life. He had his hands in four or five different businesses at once, always wanting to try something new or start something different.

It showed up in his personal life. One day, he was super dad, all in with his family. The next, he was checked out, too busy or overwhelmed to make time for any of them, including his wife.

As a result, he battled with being fully present. Even on our calls, he acted like Scrat, the little squirrel from the movie *Ice Age*. He was all over the place, literally rolling his quads out on a foam roller while we talked on Zoom. Then he'd pop a can of seltzer and start smashing a piece of grilled chicken while he walked around the room.

He was a go-getter—a high-capacity guy who seemed to succeed in everything he touched. But while his bank account was climbing, his personal life was crashing. Anxiety was eating him alive, and no amount of success could silence the internal chaos.

Then, one day, during a session, we were talking through a few of his anxiety episodes from the past week when Tori looked at him and said, "You know, I think I know what you've been struggling with the most—double-mindedness."

The second those words left her mouth, his entire demeanor shifted.

"Wow," he said, his eyes widening. "I've never thought of that before. What do you think that means?"

Sensing the light bulb moment, Tori pressed in.

"James 1:8 tells us that 'A double-minded man is unstable in all his ways,'" Tori said. "They plant one foot in and one foot out, constantly wavering. And they can't keep their balance because they're never fully committed in either direction. It's like trying to stand on two basketballs while carrying on a conversation. Sooner or later, you're going down."

I could tell he was really listening now. He stopped all his movement and leaned in.

Then she said, "I think this is why you're so distracted. Distraction is really *dis-traction*—it keeps you from gaining any traction in your life. That's why you keep ending up in the same place, stuck, with no real progress."

At that moment, I realized Tori should take the lead on our coaching calls more often! She had zeroed in on his precise struggle in just a few sentences.

As we wrapped up the call, he said he would pray about it and sit with what Tori had said. It was clear that something had clicked, and for the first time, he saw what was keeping him stuck.

He kept texting me over the next few weeks, still wrestling with the conversation.

"Man, the thought of being double-minded messed with me," he admitted. "I don't think I've ever truly decided—once and for all—that I'm done operating out of fear."

Then he added, "It was tough hearing Tori say it, but she was right—that's why I'm so distracted. And as hard as it was to hear, I think it's just what I needed. It's what I need to fix."

It wasn't an overnight transformation. It took time, effort, and plenty more conversations to help him break free from the cycle of anxiety. But I can confidently say he's in a much better place today. And—spoiler alert—when you reach the end of this book, we have a special gift for you: a full year of coaching sessions documenting the journey we took to help him break free from anxiety.

One of the foundational keys to his breakthrough was realizing that his double-mindedness was getting him off track. Everything started to change when he stopped wavering and fully stepped into faith.

"A double-minded man is unstable in all his ways" (James 1:8).

Let that verse sink in.

Unstable is an accurate word for what it feels like to live in the tension between trust and terror. You're constantly off-balance, never quite able to find solid footing.

But here's the thing—we can't live in peace and panic at the same time. Eventually, you have to decide: *Will I trust God, or keep trying to be Him?* Because when we try to control everything, fix everything, and carry everything, we're not just stressed—we're playing God.

And let's be honest, you're never going to out-God the God who made you.

Think about this: the Greek word often translated as "anxiety" in the Bible is also used for "worry," and it means "to strangle" or "to be pulled apart."[24]

Paul uses this word in Philippians 4:6, where he writes:

"Be anxious for nothing, but in everything by prayer and supplication, with thanksgiving, let your requests be made known to God ... "

The word Paul used for "anxious" or "worry" creates a powerful visual—it describes a mind being yanked in opposite directions, caught between trust and fear, faith and doubt.

Let me paint a picture that might drive this home. Imagine a rope wrapped around your neck, with one person pulling from one side and another pulling from the other. At first, it's just tension. But the more they pull, the tighter it gets—until it's strangling you.

That's what happens when you stay double-minded and let anxiety take the lead. Fear pulls from one side, and faith pulls from the other, slowly choking the life out of you. Until you decide to go all in, plant your feet firmly in faith, and stop wavering between trust and fear, you'll stay stuck in anxiety's suffocating grip.

Double-mindedness hands control over to anxiety, but single-minded faith brings peace. A single-minded person is fully committed to one goal or purpose—undistracted, unwavering, and determined to see it through. It means having one driving focus, being dedicated and resolved no matter what.[25]

I HAVE DECIDED

One of the most powerful examples of wholehearted, single-minded faith is the story behind the famous hymn "I Have Decided to Follow Jesus."

This song was my Dad's all-time favorite. And when I say favorite, I mean almost every Sunday, we belted it out like it was the only song in the hymnal.

You know the classic lyrics:

> I have decided to follow Jesus;
> No turning back, no turning back.
> The world behind me, the cross before me;
> No turning back, no turning back.
> Though none go with me, still I will follow;
> No turning back, no turning back.

Like so many of the great hymns of our faith, this song carries a powerful story.

A Welsh missionary to India in the 1880s tells the story of a family in the Indian province of Assam—a husband, wife, and their two children—who professed their faith in Christ and were baptized by him shortly after. Their decision to follow Jesus, however, came at a steep cost.

Persecution soon followed, and the village leaders, determined to make an example of them, arrested the family and demanded that the father renounce Christ.

With unwavering faith, he responded, "I have decided to follow Jesus, and there is no turning back."

The leaders responded by executing his two children right before his eyes. Still, he stood firm, saying, "The world can be behind me, but the cross is still before me."

Even in the face of unbearable loss, he refused to deny Jesus. But the demands didn't stop. Once again, they ordered him to renounce his faith.

When he refused, they killed his wife. He responded, "Though no one is here to go with me, still I will follow Jesus."

The village leaders then killed him as well. Within days of coming to Christ and within moments of one another's death, the entire family was ushered into the presence of God.

According to the Welsh missionary, when he returned to the village after the entire family was martyred, something incredible had happened—a revival had broken out. The very people who had murdered the family were now repenting and coming to faith in Christ.

The missionary shared these reports with the well-known Indian evangelist Sadhu Sundar Singh, who took the brave man's dying words and shaped them into the timeless hymn we still sing today.[26]

What an incredible testimony—a man so unwavering in his faith that nothing could shake him or make him turn back. He had already made his choice—to follow Jesus, no matter the cost.

And that's the kind of commitment that destroys double-mindedness.

This man didn't hesitate. He didn't waver between faith and fear. He didn't question whether God was still good when the pressure was on. His mind was set, his heart steady, his faith unshaken.

That's what it means to refuse to be double-minded. Anxiety thrives when we try to trust God and still hold onto control. But when we make up our minds—when we decide, once and for all, to trust God no matter what—anxiety loses its grip.

So the next time you hear "I Have Decided to Follow Jesus," remember its origin. Let it remind you that faith is a decision, not a feeling. When you stand firm in who God is and who you are in Him, you won't have to keep battling fear and doubt.

You'll finally step into peace.

CHAPTER 16

REFUSE TO ISOLATE YOURSELF

*"A friend is someone who knows
the song in your heart and can sing it back to you
when you have forgotten the words."*
–Unknown

God is not all you need.

Yes, you read that right. No, we're not being sacrilegious.

If God were *all* you needed, then solitary confinement wouldn't be one of the worst punishments imaginable. But it is.

Think about it—completely cutting someone off from human connection doesn't just make them lonely; it slowly breaks them down. Studies show that prolonged isolation leads to severe anxiety, depression, paranoia, and even hallucinations.[27] The mind starts to unravel when it has no one to anchor to.

While God is our ultimate anchor, He designed us with a specific need for others—for community, relationship, and connection.

We weren't meant to do life alone.

Look at Adam in the Garden of Eden. He had everything—a perfect, sinless world, dominion over creation, and unfiltered, direct access to God. If anyone could have thrived alone, it was him.

And yet, after declaring everything in creation "good," there was one thing God called "not good"—Adam being alone.

To fully reflect God's image, Adam needed a relationship with co-equals. God Himself exists in perfect relationship—Father, Son, and Holy Spirit. So, when He created Adam, He wired him not just for divine connection but also for human connection.

And if you want to dig deeper into how and why God created Eve—not just as Adam's companion, but with a far greater purpose—check out our book *Beauty in Battle*.

Adam needed others. And so do we.

If there's one thing we've all learned in recent years, it's this: isolation is dangerous.

We saw this play out in real-time during COVID. At first, we were told that isolation was necessary to keep us safe—but later, we saw the damage it caused. Anxiety and depression skyrocketed. People who had never struggled with mental health before suddenly found themselves crippled by fear, loneliness, and panic.

And the idea that social media and video calls were "good enough" to replace real connection? That was quickly debunked.

Social media tricks us into believing we're connected while quietly fueling the very isolation that breeds anxiety. You can have hundreds of "friends" and thousands of followers and still feel completely alone. You can spend hours scrolling, liking posts, watching stories, and reading comments—but none of it fills the need for real, face-to-face, human connection.

Social media is like junk food for the soul—it offers a quick hit of connection but leaves you starving for real nourishment. And the more we substitute screen interactions for real relationships, the more disconnected and anxious we become.

Anxiety loves isolation. It thrives in secrecy, growing stronger when no one is around to speak truth, bring perspective, or offer support. And that's why you must refuse to isolate yourself to break free from it.

Remember our coaching client from the last chapter—the one who struggled with double-mindedness? Well, one of the things that fueled his inability to go all in and make a firm decision was his increasing isolation.

The more anxious he felt, the more he pulled away from people. Instead of pushing through, he withdrew—moving his office out of a co-working space into his basement. He stopped hanging out with his friends as much because he just "wasn't feeling up to it." Even more telling? He stopped hosting Bible studies and witnessing to people—which was the opposite of his identity. Anxiety had hijacked his confidence, and isolation made it worse.

This was one of the key areas we targeted in his coaching. As he worked through fixing his wavering commitment, he started taking intentional steps to reconnect with people. He moved back into the co-working space, joined a Bible study, and started hanging out more with his buddies.

And over time? The healing process kicked in. His anxiety faded, and his energy came back. Now, he's one of the funniest guys I know. (Tori: *But he's still like Scrat from Ice Age, which only makes him funnier.*)

LET'S GO TO CHURCH

So, what about being around others makes us better, stronger, and healthier? I think the secret is found in Jesus' words:

"For where two or three are gathered in my name, there I am with them" (Matthew 18:20).

When we surround ourselves with other believers, God blesses us with a greater measure of His presence. And when we're in His presence, we receive His power.

This is why Jesus declared:

"... the gates of hell will not prevail against the church" (Matthew 16:18).

Notice, He didn't say, "The gates of hell will not prevail against a believer." He said it won't prevail against "the Church."

One person alone is a follower of Christ. But when two or more come together in His name? That's the Church. And the Church carries power.

Isolation weakens. Community strengthens. The enemy knows this, which is why his goal is always to divide and isolate—because a Christian standing alone is vulnerable. But believers standing together? That's a force hell itself can't overcome.

I love how God brings spiritual truths to life using physical examples. Jesus always did this, painting vivid pictures of the Kingdom of God using everyday things like flowers, birds, money, rocks, sand, and seeds.

The same principle applies to the power of community. One person alone can have energy, but two or more create synergy. Synergy is when exponential results happen with the same amount of effort.

Think about Clydesdale horses. One can pull up to three tons on its own. But when you hitch two together, they don't double their strength—they quadruple or even quintuple it, pulling four to five times that amount!

The same principle applies to building structures. A single wooden board can only bear so much weight. But if you double it up and attach it to another board, it doesn't just hold twice as much—it can support a load more than four times greater.

That's the power of partnership, community, and connection. Alone, we can handle some weight, but together? We are exponentially stronger!

Whether horses pulling a heavy load, wooden beams supporting weight, or people working together, the combined effort far exceeds what each could do alone.

That's the power of synergy—when two or more elements work together, their combined strength multiplies, producing far greater results than the sum of their individual efforts.

In mathematical terms, 1 + 1 doesn't just equal 2—it equals 8 (or even more)!

When people unite, incredible things can happen. That's why God had to intervene at the Tower of Babel. The people were so unified in their mission that nothing could stop them—except God Himself.

Listen to what He said:

"... If as one people speaking the same language they have begun to do this, then nothing they plan to do will be impossible for them" (Genesis 11:6).

God acknowledged the unstoppable power of synergy, a principle He created. Like any powerful force, synergy can be used for good or evil.

The power of unity is undeniable. When people work together in alignment and purpose, the impact is far greater than anything they could achieve alone.

But here's an even greater truth: When we surround ourselves with others and bring God into the mix, we don't just experience great power—we experience a power that is unstoppable, insurmountable, and Unshakeable.

We become so strong, so fortified, that not even Satan and his demons can take us down.

And the best part? We'll know it's not us. We won't be fooled into thinking we're that strong, that wise, or that capable. Instead, we'll recognize it's God's Spirit flowing through us—all of us—working together as one.

"... 'Not by might, nor by power, but by my spirit,' says the Lord of hosts" (Zechariah 4:6).

Do you want the powerful Spirit of God to help you crush anxiety, defeat overwhelm, and conquer the fears that try to take you down?

Then tap into the power of community, refuse isolation, and surround yourself with people who will build you up, speak truth, and remind you of who you are.

I want to close this chapter with a story I heard from Dr. Henry Cloud, a well-known leadership expert and clinical psychologist who has sold over 20 million books worldwide. He once shared about a fascinating study that measured the effects of relationships on stress levels, and the results were mind-blowing.

In this experiment, researchers wanted to understand how relationships impact cortisol levels, the hormone associated with high stress and anxiety (which we discussed in Chapter Three).

Here's what they did:

They took a monkey and put it alone in a cage, exposing it to intense psychological stress—loud noises, flashing lights, the whole terrifying experience. The poor thing freaked out.

While the monkey was at peak stress, the scientists measured the cortisol levels in its brain to establish a baseline.

Then, they introduced one small change.

They opened the cage door and put another monkey inside. That's it. No special training, no comforting words—just a buddy.

Then, they ran the same experiment—with the same loud noises and flashing lights—and measured the stress hormones again.

The result? The monkey's stress levels were cut in half.

Half the fear.
Half the anxiety.
Half the panic.

Simply because it wasn't alone.[28]

So, my question for you is this: Who's your monkey? Or, better yet, monkeys?

Who are you letting into your cage when life gets overwhelming? Who do you lean on when the noise is too loud, the lights are too bright, and anxiety is pressing in from every side?

Because you were never meant to fight battles alone. God designed you for community—not just to encourage and support others, but so that when life throws its worst at you, you have people who will stand with you.

Refuse to isolate yourself. Reach out. Get around people who will speak the truth when you're drowning in fear, remind you of who you are when you forget, and help carry the weight when it feels too much.

The truth is, if Adam couldn't handle it alone, you can't either.

RENOUNCE THE LIE

"Every tomorrow has two handles.
We can take hold of it with the handle
of anxiety or the handle of faith."
–Henry Ward Beecher

~~~

Time for another quick recap. Step One in overcoming anxiety is to *recognize* what's happening in the moment of attack and see the true enemy behind it all. Satan is a liar, and he uses fear to keep you trapped, but once you see him pulling the strings behind the scenes, it moves you into Step Two.

This step is where you play good defense by *renouncing* the lies you're tempted to believe in the moment of anxiety. Behind every anxious thought is a deception designed to shake our faith. Satan isn't just a liar—he's *the father of lies*. And the most effective lies are the ones that are *almost* true.

He knows how to twist reality just enough to make us take the bait, filling our minds with accusations and worst-case scenarios. But here's the key: an accusation only has power if we *agree* with it.

To renounce something means to formally reject it—to abandon it completely and refuse to let it have any power over you.

In this step, we covered five key lies that must be intentionally rejected if you want to break anxiety's grip:

- **Refuse to believe you're unsafe** – *You are not unsafe—God will protect you!*

- **Refuse to assume control** – *You were never meant to be in control—God is!*

- **Refuse to identify with anxiety** – *You are not your struggle—you are who God says you are!*

- **Refuse to be double-minded** – *You are not divided—you are single-minded in your faith!*

- **Refuse to isolate yourself** – *You cannot do this alone—you need people!*

So that wraps up Step Two - RENOUNCE. This step is all about playing good defense. Once we've stripped Satan's lies of their influence over us, it's time to go on offense!

And that leads us to the third—and most powerful—step.

Let's do this!

STEP ONE

RECOGNIZE WHAT'S HAPPENING

STEP TWO

RENOUNCE THE LIE

STEP THREE

REPLACE WITH TRUTH

CHAPTER 17

REPLACE WORRY WITH WORSHIP

*"Turn your worry into worship and
watch God turn your battles into blessings."*
–Unknown

———

It's time to go on the offensive!

We've spotted the enemy by *recognizing* that our battle against anxiety is spiritual and that Satan is behind the attack. We've defended ourselves by *renouncing* the lies he's been feeding us. Now, it's time to *replace* those lies with truth—the kind of truth that breaks chains, crushes anxiety, and sets you free once and for all.

In Step Three, we will dive into ten powerful keys—each designed to tear down the lies and replace them with God's Unshakeable truth. And we're kicking it off with the foundation of them all:

Replace worry with worship.

When you choose to worship God in the middle of your pain, watch what He does!

Worship is more than just singing songs on a Sunday morning—it's a lifestyle of honoring, adoring, and surrendering to God. At its core, worship is the act of giving God the reverence and devotion He deserves. It's a response to who He is and what He has done.

Worry focuses on *how*. Worship focuses on *who*. Worry focuses on the problem. Worship focuses on the Person—God.

When we choose to worship God in the midst of our pain, something powerful happens—He becomes bigger, and our problems become smaller.

And the doorway into worship? Prayer.

The most practical way to enter a posture of worship is to start a conversation with God. Prayer is more than just talking—it's a load transfer. When we pray, we shift the weight off our shoulders and place it in God's hands.

That's why Paul opens his famous anxiety-busting passage with this key step:

"Do not be anxious about anything, but in everything, by PRAYER ..." (Philippians 4:6).

Start with prayer. Talk to God. Transfer the load. Let it move you into worship, where anxiety can't survive.

For Tori and me, prayer is simply a conversation with God. We talk to Him like we're talking to our parents or a wise counselor. Nothing forced, just natural communication with someone we know loves us deeply and has the power to transform our lives.

One practice I've followed for years—and still do first thing in the morning to posture my heart in worship—is to kneel down, lift my hands, and speak these three simple declarations to God:

- I acknowledge Your sovereignty.
- I declare my dependency.
- I surrender my will.

That small moment of surrender shifts me from worry to worship. It sets the tone for my day, transfers the weight off my chest, and sends anxiety packing before it even has a chance to speak.

It can do the same for you. Choosing worship over worry builds your faith, brings peace, and reminds you that God is bigger than anything you will face. Even if the pain or pressure remains, He's powerful over it.

Here's the cool part—when we choose to worship instead of worry, we activate the power of the Holy Spirit in our lives.

Worship turns us from:

- Cowardly to courageous
- Weighed down to wired up
- Overwhelmed to overflowing
- Anxious to anchored

It reminds us who God is, who we are in Him, and that He is greater, no matter what we face.

Think of worship as plugging into the outlet to get the power you need. The power is there without that connection, but it cannot be accessed.

And no better story brings this principle to life than Paul and Silas in jail in Philippi.

BREAKING FREE

These two bold Jesus followers were faithfully preaching the gospel and landed in serious trouble for it. Persecution followed them everywhere. If anyone had a good reason to give in to anxiety, it was Paul and Silas. These two could have easily projected fear into the future, playing out every worst-case scenario in their minds. None of us would've blamed them if they had.

But that's not what they did.

Instead of letting fear take the lead, they stood boldly for God—no matter the cost. And cost them it did.

Due to their bold preaching in this pagan city, they were falsely accused of causing a public disturbance, beaten with rods, and thrown into prison. To make matters worse, they were secured in stocks—heavy wooden restraints fastened to the floor that locked them in place, preventing any movement.

Bruised, bloodied, and trapped in a dark, filthy prison, they could have allowed fear to overtake them. But instead of letting anxiety win, they made a choice that changed everything. Look at what they did:

"About midnight, Paul and Silas were praying and singing hymns to God, and the other prisoners were listening to them" (Acts 16:25).

In their darkest hour, they chose worship over worry. They could've easily sat in that jail cell, spiraling into fear and frustration—ruminating over how God had abandoned them, questioning why He allowed this to happen, dwelling on how unfair it all was. But they chose a better way.

They didn't wait for God to fix their circumstances before choosing peace. Unlike the disciples in the boat—who needed Jesus to calm the storm before they could find peace (Chapter Two)—Paul and Silas chose worship over worry right in the middle of their storm.

And remember how we imagined Jesus' response if the disciples had rebuked the wind and waves themselves? Now, we don't have to wonder—because we see exactly how God responds to faith like that:

"Suddenly there was such a violent earthquake that the foundations of the prison were shaken. At once all the prison doors flew open, and everyone's chains came loose" (Acts 16:26).

Their worship shook the earth. Their faith shattered their chains.

And this wasn't just a slight tremor; it was a violent earthquake, the kind you see in blockbuster action movies where buildings sway, dust fills the air, and people run for cover. I bet the whole city was in an uproar, completely panicked, trying to figure out what was happening.

But Paul and Silas? Oh, they knew exactly what was happening.

God was responding to their worship.

He didn't just gently reassure them or pat them on the back—He shook the very foundations of the earth to set His boys free. Chains snapped, and prison doors flew open. The same God who parted the Red Sea and knocked down the walls of Jericho moved heaven and earth in response to their hearts of worship.

But here's the best part of the story—because Paul and Silas chose worship over worry in their darkest hour, their freedom wasn't just for them.

Every single prisoner was set free.

All the prison doors flew open. Every chain snapped off.

Their worship didn't just break their own chains—it broke everyone's.

Can you imagine how the other prisoners must have felt at that moment? They were probably already baffled by these two new inmates singing and praising God aloud in their cell. This wasn't normal. Nobody did that in prison.

And then, suddenly, the ground shakes, the walls tremble, and their chains fall off.

I can imagine the chaos and adrenaline in that moment. As the dust settled and these stinky, sweaty prisoners looked around—cell doors open, chains lying on the ground—it must have taken a second to sink in.

And then? Total mayhem.

I picture them jumping up and down, shouting, man-hugging each other, and maybe even tackling Paul and Silas in a full-blown dogpile of gratitude! Laughter, shock, pure disbelief—because what just happened was impossible.

Maybe some of them turned to Paul and Silas, eyes wide with amazement, shouting, "Your God did this! He set us free! How can we know Him?"

That's how the jailer responded. And something tells me he wasn't the only one.

Here's the truth—the pain you're walking through, the anxiety you're battling—it's bigger than just you. God isn't wasting your struggle. He's shaping a testimony.

The mess you're in? It's becoming a message. The chains you're breaking free from? One day, you'll help others break free, too.

Your breakthrough isn't just for you—it's for them. The people who feel trapped, hopeless, and stuck in the same struggles you're facing right now? One day, your story will be the key that unlocks their freedom.

IT'S NOT ABOUT YOU

I remember God making this clear to me at the peak of my anxiety battle—when the sensations in my body were so intense, they felt like too much to bear. I was up before the sun, wrestling in prayer, begging Him to take away the pain.

And in that still, quiet moment, I felt God whisper to my spirit:

"My grace is sufficient for you, for my strength is made perfect in your weakness ..." (2 Corinthians 12:9).

It wasn't the answer I expected, but it was exactly what I needed.

I opened my Bible and read the rest of the verse.

"... Therefore I will boast all the more gladly about my weaknesses, so that Christ's power may rest on me" (2 Corinthians 12:9).

I desperately wanted God's power to rest on me, like this verse promised. But to get it, I needed to do what the next verse said:

"That is why, for Christ's sake, I delight in weaknesses, in insults, in hardships, in persecutions, in difficulties. For when I am weak, then I am strong" (2 Corinthians 12:10).

I needed to choose worship over worry right there in the middle of my pain—because that's how God's power would make me strong in my weakness.

So, I did the only thing I knew to do. I got down on my knees, right there in my room, lifted my hands toward heaven, and declared the three powerful truths from the beginning of this chapter:

- I acknowledge Your sovereignty over my struggle.
- I declare my dependence on You.
- I surrender my will regarding this situation, once and for all, to You.

Then, instead of begging God to take it all away, I thanked Him for allowing me to go through this struggle. It meant I would see His power working in me in the middle of my weakest moment.

And no sooner did I pray that prayer than I heard God whisper to my spirit:

This isn't about you. It's about others.

At that moment, I remembered the story of Paul and Silas. I knew exactly what God was telling me: the same way He was going to set me free from the chains of anxiety, He would use my story to help others break free from theirs.

I took that as a direct assignment from the Lord.

So I grabbed my phone, opened a new note, and titled it "Anxiety Notes." For the next three years, I wrote down every insight, every breakthrough, every truth that helped me overcome.

Now you're reading the result of those notes.

And as I sit here writing, thinking about you and the battle you may be fighting, I need to tell you something important.

I feel a shaking!

Your freedom is coming!

And when it does … please, no dogpiles!

CHAPTER 18

REPLACE FEAR WITH FIGHT

*"Gather up your fighting spirit,
or the disease will defeat you."*
–Aya Kito

You'll never defeat anxiety unless you muster up the warrior spirit within you.

Anxiety isn't passive—it doesn't back down just because you wish it would. It's a relentless enemy, constantly pressing, pushing, and trying to take ground in your life. And if you don't fight back, it will rule you.

This battle requires aggression. You must face your enemy head-on, sword in hand, ready to take its head off. If you don't, it will keep coming back—stronger, bolder, and more relentless each time.

If you want complete deliverance from anxiety, you've got to attack it like a warrior storming the battlefield.

It's a simple choice—when things don't go as planned or the path ahead gets dark, you either step into fear as a *worrier* or rise up in faith as a *warrior!*[29]

In the last chapter, we talked about the power of worshiping God in the midst of your pain—how it invites the Holy Spirit to break the chains that bind you and shift the atmosphere around you.

This chapter takes it one step further.

Now, we're diving into the proper posture of worship—not just hands lifted, heart open—but a warrior, sword in hand, ready to battle the enemy.

You can't approach anxiety with soft, sentimental worship songs and expect it to back down. Sure, those moments of gentle surrender have their place. That's where I started, as you saw in the last chapter.

But I didn't stay there. I got aggressive. Very aggressive.

Why? Because anxiety kept coming back. No matter how many times I worshiped or prayed, it wasn't letting up. And I wanted it to stop—once and for all.

I realized I had to approach it differently. Anxiety was coming at me aggressively, so it was time for me to fight back with the same intensity. But I wasn't able to do that until I saw a powerful truth:

Worship and warfare go hand in hand.

That truth came alive when I read the story of the Israelites taking down the city of Jericho.

TEAR DOWN THOSE WALLS

As you recall from the Book of Exodus, God's people had one mission: to escape Egypt and reach Canaan, the Promised Land. Egypt was a place of bondage, while Canaan was a place of freedom and abundance.

But between bondage and freedom, there was a battle. And Jericho was standing in the way.

The story serves as a modern-day parable for our lives. God doesn't want us to stay locked up in fear and anxiety—He has a Promised Land for our lives, a place of freedom, peace, and abundance.

The only problem was that the Canaanites were massive—like legit giants. They were fierce warriors who knew how to fight much better than the weak-sauce Israelites.

The first enemy they faced was the people of Jericho, a city with walls so thick and high they were known all over for being impenetrable. Archaeologists estimate that the city was fortified with not one but two massive walls. The outer wall was about six feet thick and 30 feet high, while the inner wall was even taller and stronger.[30]

For the Israelites, this was a humanly impossible battle. From a purely logical standpoint, there was no way in, no path to victory, and no reason to believe they could win.

Jericho stood in the way of the very place God wanted them to be. There was no going around it—only going through it. But how would they take it down?

Let's open the book of Joshua and see how it unfolded. Pay close attention to the steps they took to achieve victory!

"Then the Lord said to Joshua, 'See, I have delivered Jericho into your hands, along with its king and its fighting men'" (Joshua 6:2).

God declared victory before the battle had even begun. The walls were still standing, the enemy was still inside, and yet—God had already won the fight.

STEP 1 - Believe in victory before you see it.

Trust that God can and will deliver you from anxiety—even before it happens.

Then God gave Joshua the next instruction:

"March around the city once with all the armed men. Do this for six days" (Joshua 6:3).

The Israelites were to march—fully armed, weapons in hand, ready for battle.

STEP 2 - Get battle-ready!

Position yourself like a soldier prepared for war. Anxiety is an enemy—it won't back down unless you fight back.

Then God gave another command:

"Have seven priests carry trumpets of rams' horns in front of the ark. On the seventh day, march around the city seven times, with the priests blowing the trumpets" (Joshua 6:4).

The priests and the Ark of the Lord—which represented God's presence—were to go before the soldiers.

STEP 3 - Lead with worship!

Go into battle with God's presence at the forefront. This is a great picture of how worship and warfare go hand in hand.

Then Joshua gave a bold command:

"... Do not give a war cry, do not raise your voices, do not say a word until the day I tell you to shout. Then shout!" (Joshua 6:10).

The Israelites weren't told to shout *after* the walls fell—they were to shout *before*.

STEP 4 - Shout your victory!

Shout your war cry in faith, knowing the walls are coming down.

Now, watch what happened next.

"When the trumpets sounded, the army shouted, and at the sound of the trumpet, when the men gave a loud shout, the wall collapsed; so everyone charged straight in, and they took the city" (Joshua 6:20).

The impenetrable walls? Gone. The fortress of the enemy? Leveled.

What seemed impossible crumbled in an instant—not by human strength, but by God's power.

STEP 5 - Claim your victory!

When God declares it, it's already done. Walk in that truth.

And here we are, thousands of years later, still talking about this incredible victory.

SHOUT ... SHOUT ... LET IT ALL OUT

The story of Jericho became real to me when I realized anxiety wasn't going away. I had developed a strong habit of replacing worry with worship, and I could feel a real shift happening in my life. I was in a much better place. But something was still missing—I wasn't experiencing complete deliverance.

During this time, I found myself gravitating toward two specific songs—"Gratitude" by Brandon Lake and "Worthy of It All" by CeCe Winans.

Every morning, I'd get up early, put those songs on repeat, and let their truth wash over me. It was more than just listening—it was soaking in the reality of who God is and what He had already done.

Then, one morning, I had to take my son and nephew to the airport for an early flight. It was still dark outside, and about fifteen minutes into the drive, that all-too-familiar wave of anxiety hit me.

It was the same terrifying feeling I had been battling for months. The kind that had forced me to pull over on the side of the road before, gripped by the fear that I might pass out behind the wheel.

But this time, I couldn't stop. The boys couldn't miss their flight, and I knew I had no choice but to push through. I gripped the steering wheel, took deep breaths, and started praying—hard. I reminded myself: *I'm okay. I will get through this.*

And somehow, I did. I dropped them off, and everything was fine.

But on the drive home, as the sun began to rise and that awful, anxious feeling still lingered in my body, something inside me shifted.

It was like a fire had been lit deep in my soul. It felt like the warrior in me—the one that had been hiding in a cave—was finally storming onto the battlefield.

It reminded me of that iconic scene from *Braveheart* when William Wallace (aka Mel Gibson) rides over the hill, face painted blue, sword in hand, bellowing a war cry that shakes his army to life. That was me—except I wasn't riding into battle on a horse. I was behind the wheel of my car, driving down the highway, fed up with fear and ready to fight.

At that moment, CeCe Winans' song "Worthy of It All" was playing, and I cranked the volume as high as it would go. And right as the chorus hit, something in me erupted.

I let out the loudest shout of my life.

"YOU ARE WORTHY OF IT ALL, GOD!" I yelled at the top of my lungs.

And as CeCe kept singing, I kept shouting, "I'M SICK OF THIS! I'M DONE WITH THIS STRUGGLE! SATAN—YOU HAVE NO HOLD OVER ME ANYMORE! I AM FREE!"

I wasn't just shouting to be loud—I was declaring war.

The moment I started shouting my freedom, my body responded.

It was like a surge of strength rising up from the inside out—so powerful that I found myself pounding my fist on the dashboard, yelling at the top of my lungs:

"I'M FREE!!!" I continued. "ANXIETY, FEAR, DOUBT—YOU HAVE NO HOLD ON ME!"

I didn't just say it—I declared it. Over and over until every ounce of fear knew it had lost.

I kept going for several minutes, pouring everything I had into that moment until I was so exhausted I couldn't yell anymore.

Then, I turned the music down, let the song keep playing, and felt my body begin to relax.

At that moment, I knew I wasn't just *fighting* fear—I was *beating* it.

By the time I pulled into my driveway, I felt like a completely different person.

I'm not exaggerating—my body felt free. There was a deep sense of rest, a kind of peace I hadn't experienced in a long time. And as I stepped out of my truck, I knew I had just stumbled onto something powerful.

Worship isn't meant to be just the soft, reflective kind—where we sit, soak, and contemplate God's goodness like we're listening to a Barry Manilow ballad. Yes, there's a time for that. But that's only part of the picture.

Worship is also a weapon. It's meant to be ferocious. Loud. Unapologetic.

It's supposed to sound like a lion roaring in the face of the enemy.

Like Brandon Lake says in the song "Gratitude"—"You've got a lion inside of those lungs. Get up and praise the Lord!"

And that day, I finally let my lion roar.

Later, I learned that the Hebrew word for "shout" in the Psalms doesn't just mean "to shout" or "cry out"—it also means "to roar."[31]

Shout is not just about making a loud noise—it's a war word. It's the kind of sound that comes from deep within, shakes the ground, and prepares you for battle.

So when David tells us in the Psalms to *"shout to the Lord,"* he's not just talking about singing a little louder. He's telling us to armor up. To roar like a warrior. To be like the Israelites at Jericho, raising a war cry that brings strongholds to the ground.

And make no mistake—it wasn't just the sound of their voices that made those walls collapse. It was the power of the Almighty God roaring through their mouths.

Worship isn't a mere melody—it's a weapon. It's the battle cry that shakes the ground beneath the enemy's feet, the roar that reminds fear it has no place here. When you replace fear with fight, you stop letting anxiety call the shots and start taking ground.

The Israelites didn't whisper their way to victory at Jericho—they shouted. And when they lifted their voices in a war cry of faith, God moved.

The same happened for me. It can—and will—happen for you.

Let your worship lead you into warfare.

Don't shrink back—shout back.

Don't let fear silence you—roar in the face of the enemy.

The powerful Spirit of Almighty God isn't just with you—He's inside you. So let Him out of the cage!

And as your own life's history will prove—when God is with you, walls come down.

Worrier or Warrior—the choice is yours.

CHAPTER 19

REPLACE CHAOS
WITH CLARITY

*"The only thing worse than being
blind is having sight but no vision."*
–Helen Keller

~~~~~

Anxiety is a chaos problem. It thrives on complete disorder and confusion.

The Bible opens by setting the stage for the chaos introduced by Satan:

"Now the earth was formless and empty, and darkness was over the surface of the deep ..." (Genesis 1:2).

Darkness and chaos go hand in hand. Where there is no light, there is no clarity. There is no direction. There is no peace. In the beginning, the world was a swirling mess of disorder, a picture of what life looks like when confusion reigns.

And who is the author of that confusion? Satan. His goal has always been the same—to keep you in the dark, lost in uncertainty, overwhelmed by a sense of emptiness.

But what did God do next? He spoke.

"And God said, 'Let there be LIGHT' ..." (Genesis 1:3).

And with His words, light shattered the darkness, and everything changed.

Anxiety wants to keep you in Genesis 1:2—formless, empty, and lost in the dark. But God's plan for you is Genesis 1:3 because clarity is what moves you forward.

Our book *Brace For Impact* discusses how Genesis 1 isn't just about creation; it's about a collision—the Kingdom of Light colliding with and overcoming the Kingdom of Darkness.

I won't dive into all the incredible details here (it's well worth the deep dive), but this is what you need to know: once God's Light entered the chaos, order followed. The rest of Genesis 1 is a masterclass in how God brings structure and clarity to what was once chaotic and dark.

That's exactly what God wants to do in your life. Anxiety breeds confusion, but God's Light brings order, direction, and peace.

Satan loves keeping you in a fog because as long as you're confused, you're not moving forward. He doesn't need to destroy you if he can distract you. He knows that if you're too busy second-guessing everything, you won't be confident to step into what God has for you.

The way out? Clarity—a clear vision of what you're aiming for in life. Vision gives your mind a destination. Instead of letting anxiety toss you around like a leaf in the wind, you plant your feet, set your sights, and move forward. Because when you know where you're going, anxiety loses its ability to keep you stuck.

You can't win a battle without a clear vision of what victory looks like.

Have you ever stopped to think about what you want your life to look like five years from now? Maybe you've done it before. Maybe you haven't. When anxiety takes over, the last thing on your mind is a clear vision of the future.

Why? Because anxiety hijacks your imagination. Instead of seeing where God is leading you, all you see are worst-case scenarios. Anxiety projects fear into the future, and when fear shows up, clarity walks out the door. It's like sitting in a movie theater, fully locked into the story, when suddenly someone walks up and yanks the curtain shut. The picture was there, but now? Total darkness.

That's what Satan wants—to cut off your vision, so all you're left with is confusion, fear, and uncertainty. But God is the one who pulls back the curtain and floods your mind with light. He gives you clarity, direction, and a future worth stepping into.

EYES TO SEE

We have no better example of the power of vision than Christ's own life.

Did you know Satan tried to take him down by throwing anxiety and panic His way? Yeah, me neither—until I saw it buried in the details of what happened the night before He was betrayed.

Jesus was in the Garden of Gethsemane, pouring His heart out in prayer. He knew what was coming—the most brutal, agonizing death any human could endure. And if you read the account leading up to the crucifixion, it's clear that He was in an intense mental and spiritual battle. Yes, He was winning—but it wasn't easy.

It got so intense that He began to sweat blood drops (Luke 22:44). Luke's gospel is the only one that records this detail, which makes perfect sense because Luke was a physician. I can just picture him taking notes, making sure we'd remember how much Jesus physically endured to give us eternal life. He wanted us to see that this wasn't just emotional distress—it was a full-on, body-breaking, soul-crushing moment of suffering.

Many theologians believe the mention of Christ sweating blood wasn't just poetic language by Dr. Luke—it was an actual documented medical condition called hematidrosis. It happens when extreme stress causes the tiny blood vessels near your sweat glands to rupture, mixing blood with sweat.[32] Scientists have connected it to intense anxiety—situations of extreme fear or pressure, like what Jesus was facing on this night.

Let that sink in for a second—Jesus knows what crippling anxiety feels like. He's been there—heart racing, mind overwhelmed, body physically reacting to the weight of it all.

How does it feel to know that your Savior understands your pain? For me, that realization was a game-changer. When I was at my lowest, and the anxiety felt unbearable, remembering that Jesus Himself faced it brought a comfort I can't put into words.

But here's the question: How did Jesus get through it? What gave Him the strength to stay the course when anxiety so often derails the rest of us?

Hebrews 12 gives us the answer:

"Who for the joy that was set before Him endured the cross ..." (Hebrews 12:2).

Jesus made it through the most intense physical, mental, and emotional pain any human has ever known by focusing on the joy that was waiting on the other side.

He had a vision—a clear picture of what His sacrifice would accomplish. That vision propelled Him forward, allowing Him to see *through* the cross to the victory on the other side. And thank God He did!

Instead of letting anxiety trap Him in fear and confusion, He moved forward with clarity. He knew what He was called to do, and even under the crushing weight of it all, He walked in obedience.

And because He did, we get to live in the blessing of His unwavering clarity.

That's the power of vision.

Vision shapes your future—it defines what *could be* and what *should be* for your life.

Like Jesus, you were created with a purpose. God has placed desires in your heart; when you act on them, they lead you exactly where He wants you to go. And here's the key: the clearer your vision, the more your daily decisions will align with your purpose, keeping you on the path to peace.

Think of vision like the lid of a jigsaw puzzle. What's the first thing you do when you open the box and dump out the pieces? You look at the picture on the lid. That image gives you clarity on what you're building. Imagine throwing the lid away—how confident would you feel trying to assemble the puzzle? Frustrated? Lost? Overwhelmed? That's exactly how life feels without vision.

But when you keep the picture in front of you, everything starts to come together.

I like how one pastor said it—"The clearer the vision, the fewer the options, the easier the decision."[33]

Anxiety hates clarity, so it will do everything it can to convince you to toss the puzzle lid in the trash. Because when anxiety hits, the last thing on your mind is the powerful vision of your future.

Vision isn't just a puzzle lid; it's also fuel. It's what puts gas in your tank and gives you the energy to push through life's challenges. But without a clear picture of where you're going, you'll eventually run out of gas. And when that happens, why even get out of bed? Why go to work? What's the point? Anxiety loves that place—where nothing seems to matter, and everything feels overwhelming.

We can't count how many times we've talked with people struggling with anxiety who could barely leave their houses. And one of the first things Tori always asks them is this:

"What do you want?"

That one question helped unlock her freedom from crippling fear, as she shared back in Chapter Six. She longed to be the wife and mom she had always dreamed of becoming—but fear kept getting in the way. Still, her vision was stronger than her fear, giving her the courage to break through.

So now, let us ask you the same question—What do you want?

What is your vision for your life? Where do you see yourself; your marriage, your family in five years? Ten years?

Now go after it. Don't lose sight of it! And if you feel the light dimming, if your vision starts to fade, recognize what's happening—that's Satan, using anxiety to keep you from the purpose God has for you.

Don't let him win.

FIGHT.

Just like we talked about in the last chapter. Just like Jesus did in the Garden.

Keep your vision in front of you and FIGHT.

If Jesus made it through, so can you. Because He lives *in* you, He will fight *through* you.

In my lowest moment, when my mind and body felt like a freight train flying off the tracks, the vision of my marriage and family helped pull me through.

I kept picturing our future—taking trips together, laughing in a beach house, standing on the deck, watching our kids (and grandkids) run wild in the sand while Tori and I held hands and soaked it all in. That image kept me grounded.

Sure, I had big career goals, but in the middle of anxiety, thinking about work only made it worse. The pressure to achieve, do more, and measure up only fueled the spiral.

So I shifted my focus. My vision became my family—where I wanted to be with them, what I wanted to provide for them, and how I wanted to show up as a father and friend.

That was it. And that was enough.

And guess what? I made it through! And it was Christ's example in the Garden that helped me get there.

Like Jesus saw *through* the cross to the joy on the other side, I looked past my pain and locked onto a clear vision of what I wanted. That vision gave me the fuel to keep going, not give up, and keep fighting when I wanted to quit.

And now? I'm here. Standing in the life I once only imagined.

Oh, and also—making preparations for another family beach trip!

Speaking of which, have you ever been to Topsail Island? If not, stop what you're doing, book a trip, and while you're there, do yourself a favor and try the fish taco bowls at Shaka Taco.

Seriously. Life-changing. You're welcome.

CHAPTER 20

REPLACE GLOOM
WITH GRATITUDE

"The more grateful I am, the more beauty I see."
–Mary Davis

~

W e've shared many of the keys that helped pull me out of my funk when I was at my lowest, and we'll share several more in the chapters ahead. But if we had to pick one that stands out among them all—one that helped me flip the script on anxiety more than the rest—it was this: choosing to thank God in the middle of my pain.

Yes, I learned to choose faith over fear. I took aim at negative thoughts and replaced them with positive ones. I worshipped like a warrior in the heat of battle. And I kept my vision clear, locked in on where I wanted my life to go.

But gratitude?

That's what kept it all going.

Because, if I'm being totally honest, I didn't break free from my anxiety until I chose to thank God for it.

I know. That's a tough pill to swallow. It was for me, too. Who in their right mind thanks God for their suffering? It sounds backward—maybe even a little crazy. But it's what Paul and Silas did when they sat chained up in prison. It's what Jesus did when He chose to obey God, knowing the intense suffering ahead.

And it's exactly what happens when you choose to thank God—not just for the good, not just for the blessings, but even for the pain He's allowing in your life.

That kind of gratitude breaks chains. It lifts the gloom and sets you free.

Anxiety thrives in gloom. It dims the light, dulls the joy, and makes everything feel harder than it actually is. When you're anxious, even the brightest moments can feel overshadowed by *what-ifs*, *should-haves*, and *not-enoughs*.

Gloom is the emotional fog that keeps you stuck, convincing you that things will never change and that your past mistakes define you.

I looked up what makes a gloomy day, and I was surprised to find that it's defined by three things—all starting with "D"—just like a good ole' Baptist preacher would use in a sermon. (You know by now that I love a good alliteration to help things stick!)

A gloomy day is dark, dreary, and depressing.

Sounds a lot like anxiety, doesn't it?

And that's exactly what Satan wants hanging over your life like a storm cloud. He doesn't want your mind, body, emotions, or spirit to be filled with joy and hope. No, he wants anxiety to weigh you down, to dim the brightness of your life, and to twist the things that should bring you joy into things that bring you despair instead.

For me, this was one of the scariest parts of battling anxiety. It wasn't just the physical symptoms—the dizziness, the near blackouts, or the constant swirling in my mind. Those were bad, but they weren't the worst part.

The worst part? I couldn't feel anything.

The joy that had once defined my life? Gone. The excitement I used to have for the things I loved? Now, just emptiness.

I desperately wanted to feel joy again. I wanted to laugh, to be present, to enjoy the people around me like I used to. But no matter how hard I tried, nothing worked.

One of my greatest joys has been watching my kids grow up—being there for them, supporting their dreams, and celebrating their wins. I live for those moments—going to their games or events, cheering them on, and then going out for dinner as a family afterward. There's nothing I love more.

But when anxiety hit, I started losing that joy. I stopped wanting to go to their events. I preferred staying home rather than taking everyone out to dinner. I didn't feel like cheering anyone on in anything.

And let me tell you, there's nothing like the feeling of losing your joy. That was one of the worst feelings I've ever experienced.

Now, here's the thing—I still went to the games. I still took the family to dinner. But my heart wasn't in it like before. And I think that's an important point. Because when anxiety hits, your brain and body will try to convince you to retreat, to shut down, to stay home. But that doesn't mean you should listen.

Your family needs you. So get up, show up, and go even if you don't *feel* like it. Because sometimes, the action comes before the feeling, and the joy catches up later.

I remember begging God to restore my joy. I didn't want to go through the motions—I wanted to feel alive again. As you've seen throughout these chapters, God started to do just that.

THE POWER OF GRATITUDE

When I chose to thank God—not just for the good, not just for the victories, but for the struggle itself—it helped break me free.

Just as Paul chose to boast in his weakness, I realized I could do the same. In doing so, I discovered a powerful truth:

Strength comes through strain.

If I want bigger, stronger muscles, I have to put them under a heavy load. The same is true for our mental and emotional strength. God doesn't increase the weight in our lives because He's against us—He does it because He's for us. He allows the pressure not to crush us but to build us up.

I came to believe that God was increasing my burden because, one day, I'd need the strength to help others lift theirs. The more I thought about that, the more my perspective shifted. Instead of resenting the struggle, I started thanking Him for it because I knew it wasn't breaking me; it was building me so I could help build others.

Yeah, I had plenty of gloomy days—days where the weight of anxiety felt inescapable. But here's the truth: *gloom can't survive where gratitude thrives.*

The moment you intentionally shift your focus to what's good, true, and worth celebrating, the fog starts to lift. Gratitude doesn't ignore the struggle—it reframes it. Expressing thanks stops your mind from obsessing over what's *missing* and redirects it to what's *already here*.

Jesus showed us how to do this. At the Last Supper, knowing full well the suffering ahead, He still gave thanks (Luke 22:19). In the face of betrayal, torture, and death, He chose gratitude.

If Jesus could find something to be thankful for in the shadow of the cross, we can certainly find gratitude in the middle of our struggles. And when we do, gloom doesn't stand a chance.

Gratitude is the key to stepping into God's presence:

"Enter His gates with thanksgiving and His courts with praise ... " (Psalm 100:4).

Back in Old Testament times, the Temple—where God's presence dwelled—was surrounded by a gate. To get inside, you had to enter through it. From there, you'd step into the inner courts, where the priests carried out their work, ultimately leading to the Holy of Holies, where God's presence rested.

The Psalmist is giving us a blueprint here. He says that if you want access to God's presence—where His power, peace, and joy reside—it all starts with thanksgiving.

Thank Him for what He's done.

Praise Him for who He is.

And when you do, something happens—not just spiritually, but physically. Your mind shifts, your body responds, the weight lifts. Because gratitude isn't just an emotion—it's an entry point into God's presence.

And science is finally catching up to this truth.

When you choose thankfulness, your brain releases two powerful hormones: dopamine and oxytocin. Think of these as God-designed mood boosters—chemicals that literally help rewire your brain, heal your body, and pull you out of stress, fear, and anxiety.

- Dopamine is known as the "reward chemical." It's what gives you a sense of pleasure and motivation. When you express gratitude, your brain releases dopamine, reinforcing that "this feels good—let's do it again" response. Over time, this helps shift your brain's focus from fear and stress to joy and peace.

- Oxytocin is called the "bonding chemical." It's the same chemical released when a mother bonds with her baby or when you hug someone you care about. Oxytocin reduces stress, lowers blood pressure, and increases feelings of trust and connection. In other words, gratitude not only heals your mind—it strengthens your relationships.[34]

Gratitude isn't just about making you feel better—it's about drawing you closer to God. When you give thanks in the middle of your pain, you step into His presence. And anxiety has no place in His presence. Ultimately, stress loses its grip, and fear gets replaced with peace.

So, if you've been wondering why gratitude is such a big deal, now you know—it's not just a nice idea. It's God's design for healing, freedom, and breakthrough.

Now, I think I'll listen to a little "Gratitude" by Brandon Lake. Join me?

CHAPTER 21

REPLACE SELF WITH SERVE

*"The best way to find yourself is to lose
yourself in the service of others."*
–Mahatma Gandhi

~

We can't stand selfie culture. We say that as parents who raised four teenagers right as social media took over the world. Can we just tell you how mind-numbingly annoying it is to be standing in line at the grocery store, sitting at the dinner table, or—*God forbid*—even in church and see a kid (ours or someone else's) snap a selfie like it's their full-time job?

Seriously, who cares what you look like right now?

Apparently, a lot of people. Because within seconds, likes and hearts start rolling in, and just like that—boom—a dopamine hit. A fleeting burst of validation. But while that one-second high is taking off, so is something else: anxiety, depression, and suicide rates are soaring.

If I can dust off a term from my college psychology class—that's not just correlation; it's causation. These numbers aren't randomly moving together. They're linked. Why?

Because we were never designed to be all about ourselves.

The human heart simply can't thrive under constant self-focus. When the spotlight is always pointed inward, it turns crushing. We weren't wired to orbit around ourselves.

And it's not just selfie culture. Even in therapy culture, where the aim is healing, the constant emphasis on *my trauma, my process, my truth* can become another inward spiral. And just because it sounds more sophisticated doesn't mean it's not just as self-centered.

Don't get us wrong—we're not against therapists. There's a time and place for reflection, healing, and self-awareness. But the goal is to move *through* it, not stay stuck *in* it. Because the more you obsess over yourself, the more anxious you become. Self-focus is fertile ground for fear to grow.

There's a line from Oswald Chambers that hits this dead-on:

"The continual inner searching we do in an effort to see if we are what we ought to be generates a self–centered, sickly type of Christianity, not the vigorous and simple life of a child of God."[35]

Here's the deal—when you get caught in a loop of constant self-focus, whether it's obsessing over how people see you or overanalyzing every problem in your life, anxiety kicks into overdrive. It narrows your vision until all you can see is you—your struggles, your fears, your questions. And the more you focus on what's wrong, the louder anxiety shouts.

But here's the irony—the way out of anxiety isn't found by looking inward, but by looking outward.

Yes, Step One taught us to start by looking inward—to recognize what's happening inside so we can spot the enemy behind the attack. But that's just the beginning. You're not meant to camp out in self-awareness. You're meant to move beyond it—into purpose, into connection, into *serving others*. That's where true healing begins.

Jesus laid it out plain and simple:

"For whoever wants to save their life will lose it, but whoever loses their life for me will find it" (Matthew 16:25).

At first, this might not sound like it has much to do with anxiety—but it absolutely does. Because Jesus is pointing to the core issue that anxiety feeds on: *self-focus*. The more you obsess over protecting your life, your image, your comfort, your outcomes—the more anxious and overwhelmed you become. It's like gripping sand: the tighter you squeeze, the faster it slips through your fingers.

So what's the way out?

Let go.

Shift your focus.

Instead of being consumed by your fears and struggles, shift your attention to God and how you can reflect His love and purpose to the people around you.

Jesus shows us that the path to real peace isn't found in self-preservation—it's found in self-giving. He calls us to lose ourselves *in Him*, and one of the most powerful ways to do that is by serving others.

Look at what Jesus did the night before He was betrayed:

"He got up from the meal, took off His outer clothing, and wrapped a towel around His waist. After that, He poured water into a basin and began to wash the disciples' feet" (John 13:4–5).

Think about that—Jesus was about to endure the most painful death any human would experience, and He knew it. Yet He chose to get outside Himself and serve the people God placed in His care.

That's the model. When you stop fixating on what's unraveling in your life and start pouring into someone else's, anxiety starts to lose its power. Sure, the pressure might still linger—but it won't control you. It won't stop you from doing what's right. Fear may try to whisper, but it won't win.

Every time you choose to serve instead of spiral, you push back the darkness and make room for joy to rise.

LESS SELF, MORE SERVE

Remember our coaching client from Chapter 15? The guy who struggled with crippling anxiety and, much like Scrat from *Ice Age*, always felt like he was chasing something just out of reach—while unintentionally causing chaos around him?

I was on a call with him, and he was venting about his marriage struggles. He wanted to know why things felt off and what he could do to fix them. He said his wife was acting cold and distant, and he was at a complete loss.

"Our wives are like flowers," I told him. "If we water them, they blossom. If we don't, they start to wilt. That distance and coldness you're feeling from your wife is her telling you she needs to be seen and heard."

He paused for a second before asking, "Okay … so how do I do that?"

"Let me ask you this," I said. "On our last coaching call with you guys, we talked for 90 minutes. How much of that time do you think we spent discussing your anxiety rather than your marriage?"

He thought for a moment. "Uh … most of it, I guess."

"And over the last six months that we've been working with y'all," I said, "how much of our time has been spent helping you overcome your struggles rather than hers?"

He hesitated for a second. "A lot of it."

"Exactly," I continued. "Your wife isn't the problem. You are. You've been so consumed with your own struggles that you've lost sight of her. If you want to win her back, step outside of yourself. Shift your focus 100%

to her and your kids. Show up for them. Serve them. And watch what happens."

He took a deep breath. "Okay, I'll do it."

And I'm happy to say—he did!

A few weeks later, I got a text from him.

"Dude!" he wrote, "It's working! I should've done this sooner. I've been getting out of my basement office and actually playing with the kids— it's been awesome. I've taken my wife on a few dates, and instead of talking about my stuff, I focused completely on her. She totally opened up, and the coldness and distance are gone. This is so cool."

Then he added something even better.

"And honestly, I think it's helping my anxiety, too. I'm not 100% over it yet, but the more I get outside myself, the better my headspace feels."

"That's exactly right," I told him. "Because God didn't create you just for you—He created you for others. And the first people you need to serve are those cute little kiddos that look just like you and the amazing wife God has given you."

Replace self with serve, and watch what happens.

That's the shift. That's the breakthrough. When anxiety tells you to turn inward, the real way forward is to look outward.

STOP LOOKING AT ME

Sometimes, the issue is thinking so much about your problems that you don't pay attention to the people around you. Other times, it's the weight of caring too much about what others think. You may not be snapping selfies or chasing likes, but if you're constantly worried about others' opinions, you're still stuck in the trap of self-focus.

Anxiety and self-consciousness go hand in hand. The more you obsess over what people think of you, the worse your anxiety will get. It's like walking through life with a giant mirror in front of your face, constantly analyzing yourself from every possible angle.

Have you ever walked into a room and felt like everyone was looking at you? Judging you? Yeah, that's self-consciousness at work. But here's the truth: people aren't thinking about you nearly as much as you think they are. They're too busy worrying about themselves—just like you're worrying about yourself.

Self-consciousness is a performance mindset. It makes you feel like you're on stage 24/7, trying to live up to some imaginary audience's expectations. And the more you dwell on yourself, the more pressure you're going to feel.

The saying goes, "In your 20s and 30s, you worry about what people think of you. In your 40s and 50s, you stop caring what people think of you. By the time you're in your 60s, you realize no one was thinking about you in the first place."

There's a big difference between self-consciousness and self-awareness.

- Self-consciousness is concerned with how you are perceived.
- Self-awareness is concerned with how you impact others.

Self-consciousness traps you in fear: *What if I say something dumb? What if I embarrass myself?* It keeps you focused on yourself and lets your feelings run the show.

Self-awareness sets you free. *How can I grow? How can I be more present for others?* It shifts your focus from yourself to others and how you affect them.

The difference? One keeps your focus on yourself. The other shifts your focus outward.

And that's the real solution—stop worrying so much about what others think of you and start thinking about how you can help them.

When you focus on serving others instead of seeking approval, anxiety starts losing its power. Instead of worrying about what people think of you, you start thinking about how you can be a blessing to them. And that shift—from inward to outward—is what helps break the cycle of anxiety.

Because the truth is—*freedom isn't found in making people like you; it's found in finding ways to help them.*

We told you earlier that Tori doesn't enjoy public speaking. While she will be the first to admit it's still not on her list of enjoyable activities, she's discovered something important: the less she worries about what people think of her and the more she focuses on how she can serve them, the better she feels. (Tori: *True statement!*)

The world says happiness comes from focusing on yourself. But Jesus flipped that upside down: Real joy comes from giving, serving, and pouring into others. Funny enough, science backs this up: People who serve experience lower stress, less depression, and greater overall well-being.[36] It turns out God knew what He was doing.

So if anxiety has you stuck in your head, thinking about your own well-being, do what our coaching client did—get out of your basement and start showing up for the people in your life. Serve your family. Pour into your friends. Love the people God has placed around you.

Because at the end of the day, you weren't made to obsess over yourself or your problems—you were made to make a difference. And when you do, anxiety stops running the show.

Now take your therapist off speed dial and go live your life! And resist the urge to document it with 47 selfies.

CHAPTER 22

REPLACE BURDENS
WITH BOUNDARIES

"Boundaries define our limits and
protect our inner peace."
–Brene Brown

~

I n the last chapter, we spent a lot of time talking about serving others, but this chapter is all about balance—because if you're not careful, you can get so wrapped up in helping everyone else that you forget to take care of yourself.

"Hold up," you might be thinking. "Didn't you just tell us to stop thinking about ourselves so much and focus on others?"

Yes! But we never said to ignore ourselves completely. The goal isn't to neglect your own well-being—it's to not be so self-focused that you forget about others. You can't pour from an empty cup. If you don't care for yourself, you'll have nothing left to give the people you're trying to help.

And that's why Jesus taught balance when He gave us the two greatest commandments:

"Love the Lord your God with all your heart and with all your soul and with
all your mind ... And the second is like it: 'Love your neighbor as yourself'"
(Matthew 22:37-39).

Take a closer look at that second commandment. It comes with a built-in assumption. To love your neighbor well, you must first love yourself.

Not *instead* of yourself. Not *at the expense* of yourself. *As* yourself.

This isn't a contradiction—it's a qualifier. The best way to love and serve others is to be the best version of yourself. And that only happens when you know how to take care of yourself.

Loving your neighbor is the goal. Loving yourself is how you get there.

Think of it like football. The goal is to win the game as a team, but for that to happen, you have to take care of yourself individually—train, eat right, get rest, and stay in shape. You don't focus on yourself just for you; you do it so you can show up and play your best for the team.

And when it comes to dealing with anxiety, one of the best things you can do is create boundaries. Because some of the biggest sources of anxiety in our lives don't come from our own problems—they come from other people's issues that we've somehow ended up carrying.

If you've ever felt stretched too thin, overwhelmed by commitments, or emotionally exhausted from trying to keep everyone happy, congratulations! You're overdue for some boundaries.

A lack of boundaries is like having a front door with no lock—anyone can barge in, demand your time, drain your energy, and leave you picking up the pieces. And if you say yes to everything, eventually, you'll have nothing left to give.

And here's the thing—even Jesus had boundaries.

He didn't heal everyone. He didn't let everyone get close to Him. He didn't say yes to every demand.

Sure, He loved the masses. He taught them, He fed them, and He performed miracles for them. But when it came to deep access to His life, He drew a hard line—only 12 guys got that kind of relationship.

And even within that 12, three had a closer seat (Peter, James, and John). And even within those three, one was closest (John, the disciple Jesus loved).

If Jesus, the Savior of the world, had boundaries on His time, energy, and relationships, what makes you think you can run around with a say-yes-to-everything mentality and not crash and burn?

A huge part of anxiety comes from feeling like you have to do everything, be everywhere, and keep everyone happy. But you don't.

Not every call needs to be answered.

Not every request needs a yes.

Not every relationship deserves full access to your time and energy.

And you do NOT need to feel guilty for saying "no!"

When you start setting healthy boundaries, something amazing happens—the weight lifts. You stop carrying burdens that were never yours to begin with. You stay in your lane, focusing on what God has called you to do instead of running yourself ragged, trying to meet everyone else's expectations.

And the best part? Boundaries bring freedom!

That's right—boundaries don't restrict you; they release you. When you have clear, healthy boundaries in your life, you're free to be who God made you to be—without guilt, without pressure, and without constantly feeling drained.

Picture it this way—imagine you're in a high-rise apartment on the 80th floor in New York City. You step out onto the balcony, but there's no railing. Just an open edge and a straight drop to the street below. How free would you feel to enjoy the view? You wouldn't. You'd be paralyzed with fear, hugging the wall like your life depended on it (because it kind of would).

But the second you add a railing, everything changes. That boundary doesn't take away freedom—it gives you freedom. Now, you can step outside, breathe in the air, and maybe even lean over a little to take in the view (safely, of course—no Titanic moments, please).

One of the biggest sources of anxiety in my life? Carrying too much weight that wasn't mine to carry.

I'm a natural activator. I'm the guy who typically steps up when something needs to be done. To make matters worse, I also have a slight guilt complex (okay, maybe more than slight). So, I typically feel bad whenever someone needs help, and I can't come through.

That is, until I crashed and burned, as I shared in the introduction. I had said yes to so much that I had nothing left to give. And ironically, the very thing that made me want to help everyone ended up making me useless to everyone.

I remember Tori looking at me and saying, "Just because you *can* do something doesn't mean you *should* do something."

Shots fired.

Looking back, it seems obvious, but at the time, I had no clue that, over the years, I had given too many people way too much access to my time and energy. And it wasn't just close friends or family—it was people who barely knew me!

Whenever someone shared their dream or vision with me, I felt it was my job to help them make it happen. The next thing I knew, I had a mountain of tasks on my plate and an overwhelming amount of responsibility on my shoulders, and I was completely buried in things that had nothing to do with my actual calling.

Soon, I was overworked and overwhelmed, all because I didn't know how to say "no."

Have you ever been there?

I can't put all the blame on other people—though I'd love to. The truth is, I had a hard time saying "no" to myself and the frantic pace I thrived on. If there was a task in front of me, I couldn't sit still until I tackled it. If something lingered over my head, it felt like an annoying fly buzzing around my face, demanding my attention. I had to get it done, no matter what.

I was a mess. I couldn't say "no" to myself. I couldn't say "no" to others. As a result, I had less margin, more headaches, and a lot more frustration.

WHAT WOULD JESUS DO?

I should've taken a cue from Christ when He healed the crippled man at the Pool of Bethesda. That story, found in John 5:1-15, is fascinating.

While I won't recount it all here, the gist is this: crowds of sick, injured, and disabled people gathered around the pool, hoping to be the first to enter when the waters stirred. The word on the street was that the Spirit caused the stirring, and whoever got in first would be healed. Whether or not that was true, one thing was certain—everyone there desperately wanted to be made whole.

Then Jesus shows up—the most well-known man in Israel. He walks straight to a man who had been crippled for 38 years and asks him, *"Do you want to get well?"* (John 5:6).

The man explains that he tries to get into the water when it stirs, but no one is there to help him. So Jesus does what He loves to do—He heals him.

But here's where the story takes an unexpected turn. After healing the man, Jesus *"slipped away into the crowd"* (John 5:13). He didn't stick around to heal anyone else. (At least, not that we know of.)

Can you imagine the reaction? The other sick and disabled people must have gone wild when they saw one of their own—someone who had been there for decades—suddenly walking around completely healed. I bet they started shouting and scrambling, desperate for Jesus to come and heal them, too. Why wouldn't they?

But Jesus ... *did not.*

Can you imagine how that must have felt for the others? Some of them were probably frustrated—even angry—that the Healer didn't come back for them. I wouldn't be surprised if Jesus got a bad reputation among that crowd. But He was willing to be misunderstood to stay true to His mission.

His mission was to go to Jerusalem, to hang on the cross, and to be crucified for our sins. Healing was part of what He did, but it wasn't the whole picture.

Jesus lived a life of *"yes"* to the Father. And anything that didn't align with that *yes*—even staying to heal more people—was off the table. He knew His purpose, and He didn't waver.

What about you? Could you have done what Jesus did? Three years ago, I couldn't. And it cost me dearly. But since then, I've learned to follow His example—to set the right boundaries so I can say *yes* to what God has truly called me to do.

Here's a simple boundary hack that has helped me decide when to say *yes* and when to say *no*:

- Saying *yes* when you should have said *no* leads to **exhaustion**.
- Saying *yes* when you should have said *yes* leads to **energy**.

Your body is a great indicator, so pay attention to it. It will help guide you in setting the proper boundaries.

I'll leave you with this: people who truly love you will handle your "no" better than you think.

A few days into my battle with anxiety, I had to have a tough conversation with my twin brother. I told him I couldn't keep up the pace we'd been running for so long and could no longer be the implementor in our businesses.

He was the visionary—he'd dream up the ideas, and I'd bring them to life. But it had become too much. And I had to say *no* to the guy I literally shared a womb with.

And you know what? He was *okay* with it because he cared more about my health than the success of our business.

The people who genuinely love you? They feel the same way.

So live your life of *yes*—yes to God, yes to your purpose, yes to the things that bring life and energy. And don't let anyone guilt you for enforcing boundaries. Because if you don't, you might as well toss *"love your neighbor as yourself"* right out the window.

CHAPTER 23

REPLACE MUSING
WITH MOVING

"Life is like riding a bicycle.
To keep your balance,
you must keep moving."
–Albert Einstein

We've covered a lot so far—how to fight the battle in your mind and heart and how to start winning those fights. Now, let's shift to your body.

Because when anxiety starts creeping in—when your chest tightens, your stomach churns, and that familiar wave of panic washes over you—it's easy to get trapped in your head, overanalyzing and trying to *think* your way out of it. But often, you can't think your way out of anxiety when it's right on top of you.

Looking back at the anxiety episode I shared in the introduction—when my body started tightening up, and a wave of crazy sensations hit me—logic alone wasn't going to snap me out of it. I had to do something physical.

So, I grabbed the coldest glass of water I could find and started chugging it. I specifically remember the ice clinking against the glass and how pressing it against my forehead gave me something tangible to focus on. At the same time, I took deep, controlled breaths, doing some quick breathing exercises to calm my nervous system.

And you know what? It helped. It didn't magically erase the anxiety, but it got me out of my head and into my body—just enough to walk on stage and do what I was there to do.

At the same time, I was fighting back in my mind—focusing on truth and reminding myself *I'm okay, God's got this*. I wasn't on that stage by accident—I was doing exactly what He had called me to do. And if Jesus was right there with me, then there was no way we were going under.

I was engaging the battle on all fronts—spiritually, mentally, emotionally, and physically. It didn't happen instantly, but my body started to settle over time.

There's something about getting into your body and out of your head that anxiety can't handle. It's like trying to argue with someone while they're running a marathon—at some point, the mind has to take a backseat because the body is too busy *doing something else.*

The word *muse* means to think deeply or reflect thoughtfully.[37] It's a powerful and healthy practice when God is at the center, transforming it into true meditation.

But when anxiety takes the wheel and hijacks your brain, blaring the alarm in your body, those once-productive thoughts become a runaway train, dragging you into a downward spiral—one you can't think your way out of.

So, what's the solution when this happens? Replace musing with moving. Get out of your head and into your body.

Remember Billy Ocean's legendary 1988 hit, "Get Outta My Dreams, Get Into My Car?" As I was writing this chapter, a remix popped into my head: "Get Outta Your Head, Get Into Your Body!"

Okay, maybe it won't top the charts, but it might just save you from an anxiety spiral.

When anxiety hits, do something physical. It doesn't matter what—just move. Because the more you stay trapped in your thoughts, the tighter anxiety's grip becomes. But when you start moving, anxiety loses its power.

I LIKE TO MOVE IT

Take a page out of Fred Claus's playbook—specifically, the advice he gave Santa's head elf, Willie, when Willie wanted to learn to dance.

Fred Claus is a classic Christmas movie, starring Vince Vaughn as Santa's underachieving, screw-up brother. Fred's life is a mess, but one thing he knows how to do is have a good time. At one point in the movie, he decides to help Willie—Santa's head elf—land a date with Charlene, Santa's assistant.

The problem? Willie is completely in his own head. He's uptight, insecure, and convinced he's not good enough. So Fred teaches him how to loosen up with a dance lesson.

The music plays. Fred starts moving. Willie stands like a frozen Christmas tree and mutters, "Fred, I feel ridiculous … This is very uncomfortable for me."

Fred won't let him off the hook. He fires back, "Come on, get out of your head for a second and get into your body!"

Willie still hesitates, so Fred pushes the issue: "You know what? Stop talking with this …" (pointing to his head) "… and start talking with this …" (pointing to his body).

Then Fred lays down some wisdom: "Dancing isn't about dancing. Dancing is about connecting."

At that moment, Willie takes the advice. He gets out of his head, stops thinking, and starts moving. No, he doesn't magically become the next

Dancing with the Stars champion (no spoilers here), but for one brief moment, he lets go of his insecurities and enjoys the moment.

And that's the lesson for all of us. We can either be like Willie—stuck in our heads, overthinking everything, and standing on the sidelines—or we can get out of our heads, step onto the dance floor, and start moving. Because movement helps break the cycle. It pulls us out of our anxious thoughts and into the present moment. And that's where freedom happens.

But what does that look like in real life? How do we get out of our heads and into our bodies?

Through our own experience, we've discovered four key areas that help shift us from overthinking to actively engaging in the moment:

- Breathing – Learning to control your breath can calm your nervous system and stop anxiety.
- Nature – Getting outside, feeling the sun on your skin, and connecting with creation has a grounding effect that resets your mind.
- Exercise – Moving your body, even in small ways, releases built-in stress relievers that help you break free from anxious thoughts.
- Laughter – Sometimes, the best way to get out of your head is to laugh until your stomach hurts—it's a reset button for your entire system.

Let's look at each one of these.

JUST BREATHE

Faith Hill's hit song "Breathe" might have been written for couples, but its message is solid advice for all of us. If you want to soak in the moment, be fully present. Enjoy life instead of overthinking it—don't think; just breathe.

Breathing flushes out mental clutter and resets your system. Think of it like a sink drain—when water starts pooling, all it takes is pulling the plug for everything to start flowing out. Deep, intentional breaths work the same way. They clear the buildup of stress and anxious thoughts, sending them down the drain so your mind and body can reset.[38]

When anxiety kicks in, your breathing changes—it becomes shallow and rapid, signaling to your nervous system that something is wrong. Your body reacts as if there's an emergency. But when you slow your breath and make it deeper, you send the opposite message—one of safety, calm, and control. It's like unclogging a drain, letting the tension flow out so peace can flow in.

Remember our car analogy from Chapter Three? When anxiety is in control, your foot is glued to the gas, making everything feel urgent and overwhelming. But controlled breathing helps you press the brake. It signals to your body that there's no real danger, shifting you from panic mode to peace mode.

Dr. Daniel Amen advises inhaling for four seconds, holding for two seconds, and exhaling for eight seconds to regulate your nervous system.[39] I had to do this a lot when I had my bout with anxiety, and it helped.

NATURE BOY

One of our favorite date spots is downtown Davidson, NC, home of Davidson College—also known as the place where Stephen Curry became a hoops legend. If you ever sign up for one of our marriage intensives, there's a good chance we'll bring you there.

Davidson is the perfect blend of old-town Americana with a laid-back, outdoorsy college vibe. The other day, we were wandering through one of the boutiques and saw a shirt that said, "Hike More. Worry Less." And honestly? That might be some of the best anxiety advice out there.

For almost 20 years, we've been walking that campus, hiking the trails in the woods behind it, and soaking in the stillness. There's nothing like setting up our hammocks, kicking back, and just listening to the trees sway in the wind.

Getting outside and into nature was one key way I healed from anxiety. Each morning, I'd step outside, feel the cool air on my face, listen to the leaves rustling, and let the gentle wind remind me that I was connected to something bigger than my fear. In those moments, I felt God's presence more clearly than ever.

It reminded me of Fred's advice about dancing—"It's not about dancing, it's about connecting." The same is true for getting outside. Stepping into God's creation isn't just about being in nature but connecting with the One who made it.

Why does it work? Because you were created by Him, too. The same Father who spoke the mountains into existence, painted the sky, and filled the air with the scent of pine is the One who created you. No wonder being in nature feels grounding—it's a family reunion with creation.

Science supports this. Nature immersion therapy has been proven to reduce anxiety, lower stress, and improve mental well-being.[40] It turns out that the best remedy for an overwhelmed mind might just be to step outside.

Dr. Andrew Huberman, from the Stanford School of Medicine, explains that anxiety narrows your focus, intensifying the feeling and keeping you locked in a loop. But stepping into nature engages what he calls "panoramic vision," expanding your perspective and helping your brain shift into a state of calm and healing.[41]

HIT THE GYM

No, you don't need to start deadlifting like a bodybuilder, but you do need to get your heart rate up. Everyone knows exercise is good for you, so we won't spend too much time stating the obvious.

But here's the deal—movement matters. Exercise triggers endorphins, those feel-good chemicals in your brain that boost your mood and act like natural painkillers. And if that wasn't enough, regular movement helps you sleep better, builds confidence, and gives anxiety less room to operate.[42]

Exercise is a triple threat against stress. So, whether it's a walk, a bike ride, or dancing in your living room like nobody's watching—just move.

Numerous studies have shown that exercise works as well as, if not better than, antidepressants and has zero side effects. Consider replacing the pills with plyometrics!

HUMOR ME

Laughter might just be the best antidote for anxiety we've ever found. A good, gut-busting laugh can get you out of your head and into your body faster than just about anything else. In my darkest moments, there were times when Tori would throw on a clip from one of our favorite comedians—Nate Bargatze, Tim Hawkins, or Sebastian Maniscalco—and within minutes, I'd be laughing so hard that I completely forgot I was struggling with anxiety.

Laughter is built-in stress relief designed by God Himself. When you laugh, you inhale more oxygen, engage your heart and lungs, and trigger a flood of endorphins—just like what happens when you exercise. It's like hitting a reset button for your nervous system, except you're having a great time instead of sweating at the gym.

And here's the wildest part—laughter actually flips your stress response on, then shuts it right back off. It's like a reset button for your nervous system. When you laugh, your body briefly activates its fight-or-flight mode, but instead of spiraling into anxiety, it follows up with a full-body shutdown of stress. Your muscles relax, your heart rate slows, and your brain floods with feel-good chemicals that scream, "All is well!"[43]

So, if you're feeling overwhelmed, find something to laugh about. It might be the easiest (and most fun) way to kick anxiety to the curb.

Dr. Archibald D. Hart, a pioneering psychologist and author of *The Anxiety Cure*, knew the power of laughter in battling anxiety. His advice? "Avoid seriousness." Not because life isn't serious, but because taking yourself too seriously only fuels anxiety. He explained that humor boosts the brain's natural tranquilizers, helping to release both physical and emotional tension.[44]

In other words, laughter isn't just fun—it's therapy. So watch a funny show, swap ridiculous stories with friends, or just embrace the awkwardness of life and laugh at yourself. The more you incorporate laughter into your daily routine, the more you'll rewire your brain for joy and kick anxiety to the curb.

Here's the deal—when you replace musing with moving, you tap into your body's God-given ability to fight anxiety. You weren't designed to stay stuck in your head, overthinking yourself into a frenzy. God built your body to help you heal, so use it!

Take some deep, slow breaths and feel the tension melt away.

Step outside, soak in creation, and reconnect with the One who made it all.

Get your heart pumping and let all that stress shake loose.

And most importantly—laugh. Hard. Like full-on, ugly laugh if necessary.

Because when you do, you won't be that person standing awkwardly on the sidelines, wondering if you should step onto the dance floor. Nope. You'll be out there, breaking it down like you're back at senior prom— except this time, without the bad hair and crazy fashion. Maybe.

CHAPTER 24

REPLACE CONTEMPT WITH COMPASSION

"Talk to yourself like someone you love."
–Brene Brown

~~~~~~~~~

As you've probably figured out by now, anxiety doesn't ease its way in. It barges through the door and takes over. It wants to hijack your thoughts, call the shots, and put fear in charge instead of faith.

But if you're going to stop that hijack—and take back control—you'll need something that most of us overlook: compassion. Not just for others, but for yourself.

The Bible tells us to be kind and compassionate to one another. But have you ever considered that this includes being kind and compassionate to yourself?

If you've ever struggled with anxiety, you know those voices in your head aren't exactly full of grace. They're ruthless. They don't just criticize—they berate and belittle you, tearing you down in ways that make every playground bully look nice.

I read a quote that captures this idea: "Anxiety is basically a conspiracy theory you wage against yourself."[45]

To put it another way—anxiety is a straight-up bully.

Think about it. A bully's entire strategy is built on fear, intimidation, and making you believe things about yourself that aren't true. Anxiety does the same thing. It shoves you into a corner, screams at you, and convinces you that you're not good enough, not strong enough, and never going to break free.

And just like a schoolyard bully, anxiety thrives when you don't stand up to it. The more you listen to it, the louder it gets. The more you believe it, the stronger it becomes. But here's the thing—bullies are cowards. The moment you stop playing their game, they start losing their power.

So, instead of beating yourself up for struggling with anxiety, try something radical—stand up to it while showing yourself compassion. Anxiety already plays rough. Don't help it do its job.

We've talked about having a fighter's mentality when it comes to anxiety, but that doesn't mean beating yourself up when you get knocked down. A real fighter doesn't waste energy shaming themselves for falling—they get back up and keep going. And so should you.

Imagine walking up to your 8-year-old self—overwhelmed with anxiety, scared, confused, and trying hard just to hold it together. Would you yell? Shake your younger self and demand, "Snap out of it"? Of course not. You'd kneel down, look into those innocent eyes, and speak compassionately. You'd offer reassurance: "You're safe. You're strong. And you're not alone."

So why don't we do that for ourselves now?

It's time to stop beating yourself up for struggling and start building yourself up instead. Treat yourself with the same kindness and encouragement you'd give to your 8-year-old self.

Because the words you speak to yourself matter.

LIVING A REALITY

We know a thing or two about dealing with bullies. We've learned that when you take a stand, you need voices of encouragement in your corner.

You may have heard the story of how my brother and I lost our HGTV reality show back in 2014 because a liberal activist group out of California didn't like our public stand for life and marriage. Our beliefs aligned with biblical values, not the shifting opinions of culture—and that was enough to put a target on our backs.

At the time, HGTV had big plans for us. They had hired us at the same time as Chip and Joanna Gaines, intending to build both families into cornerstones of the network. But when the backlash came, everything changed.

Six weeks into a ten-week film shoot, just as the show's commercials started airing, that activist group turned up the pressure and demanded HGTV pull the plug on our show.

The execs at HG called to give us a heads-up. But they assured us we had nothing to worry about. They knew we were Christians, and they weren't buying into the false online narrative that was smearing us for holding biblical views.

That activist group wasn't happy with HGTV for sticking with us, so instead of backing off, they did what bullies do best—they doubled down.

They crafted a fake news story about David and me, twisting our words, misrepresenting our beliefs, and making us sound like dangerous extremists. It was a total hit piece designed to bully HGTV into submission.

This was Cancel Culture before it became a popular hashtag.

They blasted the story to a bunch of media outlets, got their activist friends on board, and within hours, social media was on fire with news that HGTV had hired the "radical, whacko" Benham brothers.

The next day, our phones rang—three HGTV executives in full-blown panic mode. There was no small talk, no buildup—they got straight to the point.

"Guys, we're canceling the show!"

We weren't shocked. We saw it coming.

Growing up, we watched our dad—a pastor and a pro-life leader—get bullied constantly for his bold stand on the sanctity of life. We knew things get heated when you take a public stand for biblical values. And now, it was our turn.

So, instead of pushing back, we just thanked them.

"We get it," we said. "We know you guys believed in us. The Bible says all things work together for good, so we trust that God will use this for something bigger. We just want to thank you for standing up for us and trying to make it work."

One of them paused for a moment, then said, "Wow. I didn't think I would be speechless on this call."

We told them, "You guys got bullied into this. We know you wanted to stick with us. But there's a Goliath in culture right now—an agenda that demands silence from Christians—and we're not about to back down to it."

We hung up the phone, and that was it. Just like that, the show was over.

Word spread like wildfire. Within hours, our phones were blowing up with interview requests, and before we knew it, we were on more talk shows and news stations than we could count.

From that moment on, David and I knew our mission had shifted. What started as a reality show about our real estate business had turned into a fight against a cultural bully—one that demands conformity from men and women of faith.

And fight we did.

Here's the craziest part of the story, at least for me. I realized the biggest bully wasn't the one I was battling publicly. The real bully was the anxious thoughts I was battling privately.

I remember our very first interview with Erin Burnett on CNN. It was a live shot, which meant we were sitting in a tiny, dark room in Charlotte with two chairs and a single camera pointed at us. You can't see the interviewer. You just hear their voice in your earpiece while staring directly into the camera: no facial expressions, no body language, no way to tell how your words are landing—just talking into the abyss, hoping you're making sense.

I was nervous driving to the studio that night. And, of course, the more I thought about it, the worse it got. Anxiety isn't exactly known for staying quiet when it sees an opportunity. It pounced.

We walked into the studio, and the second I stepped through the door, the voice in my head went from whispering to full-on screaming.

"You can't do this! You're going to embarrass yourself! You have no business being on a show like this—this is for smart people!"

And just like that, anxiety went from lurking in the shadows to trying to shove me off a cliff.

I took a few slow, deep breaths, got myself under control, and sat in the chair beside my brother. (This was several years before I experienced full-blown anxiety attacks.)

It was dead silent.

At this point, we had become the No. 1 story on Facebook worldwide. The media hype was insane. Half the world loved us. The other half wanted us gone.

And now, we were about to go live.

We felt totally alone—like we were standing in the middle of a battlefield with no backup. We'd never faced an attack like this before. Sure, we had told HGTV we weren't backing down and that we'd stand firm against the cultural bully. But when the moment actually came to take that stand, it was a real fight to follow through on our word.

We did the interview. The host came at us hard, and we had to defend ourselves. It wasn't pretty. It wasn't polished. And honestly? It didn't go well. We walked out of that studio feeling like we just got our butts kicked.

I remember getting home that night, feeling completely defeated. I walked in like a whipped puppy, replaying every word, every awkward moment, every missed opportunity.

And those voices that had been screaming at me before? Now, they felt confirmed.

"You had no business being on that show. You embarrassed yourself in front of millions. You're a total failure. You're not the guy for this job."

At that point, I don't even think it was anxiety doing the talking anymore—it was me.

I had fully bought into the lie and wanted nothing to do with another interview—ever. But that wasn't an option. We already had a full lineup waiting for us, including more rounds on CNN the next day and FOX News primetime that night.

The first person to meet me at the door when I got home? Tori. She wrapped her arms around me and said, "I'm so proud of you."

I shook my head. "We bombed! It was terrible. And it's only going to get worse."

I could feel anxiety's weight pressing in. "Those CNN hosts are coming for us tomorrow. They hate everything we stand for. And to be honest? I'm scared to death."

Projected powerlessness on display.

Tori didn't flinch. She hugged me again and said, "Everything in your life has prepared you for this. I've watched you go through battles before. I've seen you stand for what's right. This is scary, no doubt, but God made you for this moment! You've got this, and I'm so proud of you."

When she said those words, I felt something lift. It was like my body physically responded to her encouragement. Her warm hug, steady voice, and unwavering belief in me reminded me that no matter what happened, I wasn't alone.

A few months later, we completed our 200th one-on-one interview. And with each one, that bully in my head got weaker and weaker—until one day, he stopped showing up.

Looking back, I can't help but appreciate how Tori handled that moment. She didn't scold me for being anxious. She didn't tell me to *suck it up* or *get over it*. She met me where I was, wrapped me in compassion, and spoke life into me. She put courage in my heart.

And that's exactly what the word "encourage" means—*to make courageous*.

But here's the thing: you don't just need someone else to encourage you; you need to learn how to encourage yourself.

If Tori had berated me that night, it would've crushed me. But the truth is, that's how most of us talk to ourselves when anxiety hits.

We tear ourselves down. We let that bully in our head run wild. We pile on guilt, shame, and self-doubt until we can barely move.

It's time to replace contempt with compassion.

The next time anxiety comes at you, speak to yourself the way Tori spoke to me.

"This is tough, but you were made for this."
"You've been through hard things before, and you'll get through this too."
"You've got this. God is with you."

Because here's the truth—if you wait for someone else to encourage you, you might be waiting a long time. You have to be your own encourager.

And the best way to do that? Fill your mind with truth from Scripture—God's own words of encouragement to you. But it's not enough to just read it. You have to speak it over yourself.

That bully will come back—bullies always do. But when you start speaking life over yourself, it doesn't stand a chance.

CHAPTER 25

REPLACE SUCCESS
WITH SURRENDER

"The harder you work, the harder it is to surrender."
–Vince Lombardi

~~~~

I like Coach Lombardi's quote above. And I get what he's saying—work hard, never quit, push through no matter what. That mindset is great in sports, business, and many areas of life.

But when it comes to anxiety? You've got to be careful what you're working toward because ambition and anxiety are linked.

I can't count how many times I've coached entrepreneurs, high achievers, and go-getters who were crippled by anxiety. Why? Because they let ambition spin out of control. Their desire to accomplish big things, build something great, and conquer the world pushed them to press the gas and rip the brake pedal clean off.

It works for a while. But eventually, the never-ending pressure to perform catches up with them. And when it does, they crash and burn—hard.

And the cruel irony? The very thing they were chasing—success—is what took them out.

And this isn't just an entrepreneur problem.

We all have dreams, goals, and visions of what we want to accomplish. But if we're not careful, we jump on the hamster wheel, running as hard and fast as possible, chasing something that always seems just out of reach.

Until one day, we're not thinking about conquering anything. Instead, we're wondering why we feel so conquered.

Here's the key—*we are not meant to find security in success; we are meant to find it in surrender.*

Success is a moving target. It's never enough. There's always another milestone to hit, another level to reach, another goal to check off. And if you tie your sense of worth, peace, and security to success, you'll always be one step away from feeling like a failure.

But surrendering to God means trusting His process. It means embracing His pace of growth instead of trying to force our own. It means recognizing that our value isn't tied to our achievements but to who we are in Him.

Surrender isn't easy. Letting go feels unnatural if you're wired to chase big goals, push forward, and make things happen. But here's the truth: Surrender isn't giving up; it's giving over. It's shifting the weight off your shoulders and placing it where it belongs—on God.

Because when your security is in His hands, not your hustle—that's when real peace begins.

One of my favorite quotes is from Oswald Chambers:

"Focus on depth and let God handle your breadth."[46]

That one line perfectly captures the heart of surrender.

When you release the results of your life into God's hands, allowing Him to determine how far, how high, and how wide your influence grows—instead of striving to make it happen yourself—you unlock a whole new level of peace.

And I know this from experience.

Looking back at my battle with anxiety, I started to see a pattern. The relentless pace I kept in business wasn't just a contributing factor—it was fueling the fire. I felt like a freight train with no brakes, barreling forward at full speed. And here's the scary part—I didn't want to stop. I had fun building businesses, speaking on stage, and writing books … until I didn't.

PUSH THE BRAKES

Shortly after my biggest meltdown, I had a moment of clarity as I took time off to recover at home. I was sitting on the couch with Tori, enjoying a rare moment of stillness, when out of nowhere, a thought hit me—*I need to start writing a book about this anxiety stuff!*

The minute that thought hit my head, I started feeling anxious about the need to write it *now*! My heart began to race, and those same anxious feelings I had been battling came rushing back. What had been a peaceful, Level One moment instantly cranked up to Level Three, all because my brain decided to fast-forward to the million things I needed to do instead of just being present with my wife.

I told Tori about it, and without missing a beat, she reminded me, "You are not supposed to be doing anything right now. You need to heal from the frantic pace that got you here in the first place."

"Oh, and by the way," she added, "you've written six books in six years. Maybe that pace has something to do with why I'm here trying to rehabilitate you!"

Shots fired. But she wasn't wrong.

So, I took her advice. I shut my brain off to my need to accomplish and allowed myself just to be. And you know what? It felt freeing. I realized that I didn't need to rush to *write* the book—I needed to *live* the book I wanted to write.

As I reflected on why I had this constant drive to do big things, I traced it back to my college years at Liberty University. One of the big themes there was this: "God wants to use ordinary people to do extraordinary things." And I took that message to heart. I wanted to go big for God.

But the more I focused on doing great things for God, the more I found myself moving at a breakneck pace, chasing massive goals and huge dreams. I wanted to see people come to know God, help them grow in their faith, and make a real impact for the Kingdom.

All of these were *good* things. But it shows you how sly Satan is. He doesn't just tempt us with bad things—sometimes he takes our good desires, even our God-given desires, and twists them just enough to send us spinning out of control.

If we're not careful, our passion for doing things for God can push us past the limits He's set for us. And when that happens, anxiety isn't far behind.

Here's the crazy part—several of my friends who went to LU were also battling anxiety. I'm not blaming our alma mater, but it became clear that a lot of us got so caught up in trying to change the world for Christ that we let our own worlds start falling apart.

We needed to take a page from Oswald Chambers' book—stop obsessing over breadth and start focusing on depth. Because the more we chase the size of our dream, the more it starts controlling us.

In that season of forced stillness, I finally understood that God wasn't asking me to stop dreaming or working hard. He was asking me to stop striving and start surrendering.

We've learned that a relentless drive for success can quickly become a deep desire for approval. We want people to think well of us, respect us, and never see us as failures. In a way, we're chasing validation, hoping the world will hit the "Like" button on our lives.

And here's the danger: the more you chase success, the more you elevate "likes" over "lives." Instead of serving and loving the people God has put in your path, you start serving an image—an idea of how you want to be seen.

I recently heard Dr. Chuck Swindoll tell a story about a woman stuck in this exact trap on his podcast, *Insight For Living*.

After her husband passed away, she was left to raise several children on her own. She gave it her best shot, but anxiety started creeping in—not just over the challenges of parenting, but over how she looked to the outside world. She wanted everyone to see her as strong and capable— like she had it all together.

As a result, she wouldn't let her kids go to church or school without the perfect outfit. She stressed over their behavior in public, terrified they'd embarrass her. She worked overtime to make sure everyone around her saw that she was in control—that she was okay.

But underneath it all? She wasn't okay. The harder she worked to make her kids into perfect little specimens, the worse her anxiety became. No matter how much effort she put in, it was never enough.

Until one day, she hit a breaking point. Anxiety came flooding in, and she knew she had to make a change.

She finally let go—not just surrendering to God, but releasing the pressure to live up to the impossible standard in her mind. She even told God, "If I look like a failure, that's okay with me."

And in that moment? Her anxiety was gone.

Just like that, she was free.

A quote I read summarizes her story perfectly—"I just give myself permission to suck … I find this hugely liberating."[47]

We could not agree more.

It's amazing what happens when you replace success with surrender; when you stop white-knuckling control and allow God to set the pace; when you move ambition out of the driver's seat and let acceptance take its place.

Does God use ordinary people to accomplish extraordinary things? Absolutely. He can, and He will.

But if you truly want freedom from anxiety, don't focus on doing the big things. Focus on being faithful in the little things.

Because here's the truth:

God doesn't just use ordinary people to do extraordinary things—He uses extraordinary people to do very ordinary things.

And you are one of those people.

CHAPTER 26

REPLACE PANIC
WITH A PROCESS

"The process is the foundation for success.
Trust it, embrace it, and let
it guide you to success."
–John Addison

There's a saying in the military: "You don't rise to the occasion; you fall to the level of your training."

When a soldier steps onto the battlefield, panic is not an option. Every movement, every reaction, every decision has already been rehearsed a thousand times. Why? Because when the pressure is on and chaos erupts, there's no time to think. The soldier doesn't rely on feelings; they rely on their training.

And that's what you need to overcome anxiety. That's why we're closing this book with the principle that combines everything you've learned into one powerful strategy—a process to help set you free.

In the heat of the moment, you won't magically rise with courage and clarity. You'll default to whatever process you've trained yourself to follow.

That's why having a battle plan in place before anxiety hits is crucial. If you don't have a process, you'll scramble. You'll react out of fear, let emotions drive your decisions, and most likely spiral deeper into anxiety.

But when you've trained yourself to follow a process—one that's simple, clear, and effective—you won't freeze; you'll act.

Just like a soldier doesn't wait for war to start training, you can't wait until panic hits to figure out what to do. You prepare now. You train now. Because when the moment comes, you don't want to fall into fear—you want to rise with a plan.

The three-step plan we've shared with you is the process, and it's powerful. But only if you practice it until it becomes second nature. And that will take discipline.

Discipline is doing what you *don't* want to do to accomplish what you *do* want. Your natural instinct is to give in to worry, doubt, and fear. But instead of following that old pattern, you can train your mind to take a different path—*recognizing* the enemy behind the attack, *renouncing* the lie he wants you to believe, and *replacing* it with the truth that sets you free.

It won't feel easy at first. We know that full well. But the more you push through and do the hard thing, the easier it gets. Over time, this process won't just be something you do—it will become who you are.

Do you know how you can tell when you've been fully trained? When you no longer need discipline to do the thing anymore, because it's now your default mode.

And that's where you're headed.

Trust us—what's on the other side of this process is worth it. If you commit to these three steps, it can rewire your brain.

Dr. Caroline Leaf explains that your brain constantly rewires itself based on what you think most. It's called neuroplasticity, and it means that your thoughts aren't just thoughts; they're actually shaping your brain. So when you replace anxious, negative thinking with truth, you're not just making yourself feel better in the moment—you're rewiring your brain to think differently.[48]

The more you interrupt anxious thoughts and replace them with truth, the stronger those new pathways become. Over time, peace becomes your default instead of panic. But it doesn't happen overnight. The key is consistency.

FROM OLD TO NEW

Seeing how science is finally catching up with the Bible is amazing. Romans 12:2 literally describes neuroplasticity long before modern research ever did:

"Do not conform to the pattern of this world, but be transformed by the renewing of your mind ..."

The Greek word for "transformed" here is "metamorphosis"—which means "a complete change in form or nature, either by natural or supernatural means."[49]

In other words, God designed your brain to be rewired. That's what transformation is. You're not stuck. You're not doomed to think the same anxious thoughts forever. You can change. Science now confirms what Scripture has said all along—what you focus on shapes who you become.

The same process takes a caterpillar and turns it into a butterfly. When the cocoon forms, the caterpillar's DNA dissolves, and an entirely new set of DNA activates—butterfly DNA.[50] It's not just a small change; it's a complete transformation. Science still can't fully explain how it happens, because it's supernatural.

And here's the best part—God can do the same thing in you.

The same God who designed a crawling caterpillar to become a soaring butterfly can turn your fear, doubt, and anxiety into peace, confidence, and freedom. But just like the caterpillar has to go through the cocooning process, you have a part to play, too.

You have to renew your mind.

Renewal is all about taking off the old and putting on the new. Like Tori removes her old fingernail polish before she applies the new, you have to remove old thoughts (based on lies) and replace them with new thoughts (based on truth).

That's why renewing your mind is a daily process. Over time, as you consistently fill your mind with truth, you'll start to think, live, and respond like the new you.

That's what our 3-step process is all about. When you *recognize* the enemy behind the attack, *renounce* the lie he wants you to believe, and *replace* it with truth—that's renewal in action. And God's promise is clear: this process will transform you.

But here's something crucial to understand—our plan isn't just for the moment anxiety strikes. It's not just a rescue strategy when you're under attack. It's also a training plan to strengthen your mind before the battle begins.

Just like a soldier doesn't wait until the battle begins to learn how to fight, you can't wait until anxiety strikes to start practicing *Recognize, Renounce, Replace.* If you want to stand strong in the heat of the moment, you have to train before the pressure is on.

This means consistently running through the three steps—even when you're not struggling. The more you Recognize the enemy's lies, Renounce them, and Replace them with truth in your everyday life, the more automatic it becomes.

To help you lock in this process and make it second nature, we've created a simple exercise that will train your mind before anxiety has a chance to take hold. Think of it like strength training for your brain. The more you practice, the stronger you get. Over time, truth will become your default, and when anxiety tries to creep in, you'll already have the right weapons in place to shut it down.

EXERCISE:

- **Write down three things** that trigger anxiety for you.
- **Write down the lie(s)** you're tempted to believe in each moment.
- **Find a Bible verse** that directly counters each lie.
- **Write a personal declaration** that takes the truth of that Scripture and applies it to your life.
- **Memorize** your verse and declaration.
- **Speak them out loud** every morning, every night, and whenever you're anxious.

Throughout the day, when you're not feeling anxious, let your mind dwell on these powerful truths. This daily exercise will help rewire your brain. As you consistently replace lies with truth, your mind will transform, and anxiety will lose its grip.

And here's the best part—when fear does show up, when anxiety tries to crash in on you, these verses and declarations become your lifeline. They're the specific truths that will replace the lies you're tempted to believe at that moment. They'll become the weapons you'll wield until peace takes over and anxiety fades.

In time, truth will become your automatic response, new neuropathways will be created, and you will be free.

BEND YOUR KNEES

Let me share a personal example of how this played out in my life. If you remember, we talked about how trauma comes in many forms—and one of its lasting effects is that it leaves triggers behind. These triggers don't just disappear with time; they often stay with us for life.

When I was 12, my school switched to uniforms, and they picked a handful of students to model them for all the parents at a big event. Apparently, they thought I had the look for it, but interestingly, they didn't pick my twin brother. This erased all doubt as to who the better-looking brother was. But I digress.

The night of the event, moments before I was about to walk on stage, my dad—always full of wisdom—offered some well-meaning but wildly unhelpful advice.

"Hey, Jeets," he said (his nickname for me). "When you're up there in front of all those people, make sure you bend your knees. We learned to do that in the military, so guys wouldn't pass out from standing still too long."

Just what every 12-year-old needs to hear right before stepping in front of a packed crowd—"Don't lock your knees, or you might pass out!"

I know he meant well, but how did that affect me? As a scrawny, not-even-close-to-hitting-puberty kid just trying to make it through middle school without embarrassing myself, it scared the life out of me.

Before that moment, passing out on stage had never crossed my mind. But that night, it was all I could think about.

I stood up there, completely panicked. *Are my knees bent enough? Should I go full squat? Wait, am I swaying? What if I actually fall over in front of EVERYONE?!*

One simple comment turned an uneventful moment into a full-blown crisis in my mind.

Thankfully, I made it through the night without face-planting on stage— and since I didn't have to stand in front of crowds much as a kid, I didn't think about it again. I figured it was just a weird moment, nothing to worry about.

Little did I know that seemingly small event had buried itself deep in my subconscious. It had left a mental and emotional imprint, just waiting for the perfect moment to resurface.

And for years, it stayed hidden. I moved on and never gave it a second thought.

Until I was 46 years old, standing backstage at a pro-life event in Vidalia, GA, where his words would come back to haunt me.

I told you about this night in the introduction—when anxiety jumped on me and threw my body into a full-blown panic.

And can you guess the one thing running through my mind?

The exact same thing I was thinking 34 years earlier—*Just don't pass out!*

What I didn't realize was that the unintentional trauma from that night long ago had buried itself deep in my subconscious. I had no idea it was even there. But the moment anxiety hit me, that old fear came roaring back.

Suddenly, my biggest worry wasn't the speech, the crowd, or the event itself. My greatest fear was the same one I had as a kid—passing out in front of everyone.

That night in Vidalia, I wasn't 46-year-old, confident, I-know-who-I-am Jason.

I was 12-year-old, terrified, scared-out-of-my-mind Jason.

Now you see what was happening inside my brain—the deep-seated fear I had to work hard to rewire and replace with truth. It wasn't easy, but the 3-step process in this book is how I did it. And the exercise in this chapter? That's how I locked it in.

When it came to speaking on stage, here's how I put this exercise into action:

- Event – Standing on stage in public triggered anxiety.
- Lie – You're going to pass out in front of everyone.
- Verse – *"I can do all things through Christ who strengthens me"* (Philippians 4:13).
- Declaration – "I am called by God to strengthen believers. I have the peace and power of God when I stand on stage and walk in obedience to my calling."

I stand on stages all over the country now. And every once in a while, a fleeting thought tries to sneak in—that old trigger, tempting me to step onto the stage as 12-year-old Jason.

But I know the truth. And I've repeated Recognize, Renounce, Replace so many times that it's become second nature. My brain has been rewired and I am free.

Here's the best part—if it worked for me, it can work for you.

So here's the question—will you keep crawling through life like a caterpillar? Or will you let God give you wings?

Because you weren't made to stay on the ground.

You were made to fly.

REPLACE WITH TRUTH

*"And then you will know the truth,
and the truth sets you free."*
–Jesus Christ

———

Step One in overcoming anxiety is to *recognize* what's happening in the moment of attack and see the true enemy behind it all. Satan is a liar, and he uses fear to keep you trapped.

Step Two is where you play good defense by *renouncing* the lies you're tempted to believe in the moment of anxiety.

Step Three is where you go on offense and *replace* those lies with truth. And when you build your life around truth, it will set you free.

As you anchor yourself in worship and step into anxiety with a battle-ready mindset, it doesn't stand a chance.

When you shift your focus beyond fear, fix your eyes on the joy ahead, and walk in gratitude for all God has done, anxiety loses its grip.

The more you pour into others while maintaining healthy boundaries, the more you'll experience a freedom you never thought possible.

Getting out of your head and into your body grounds you in the presence of the very God who created you.

When you show yourself compassion, calm your restless striving, and surrender fully, peace will flood your heart and mind.

And when you've trained yourself to follow a simple, clear, and effective process, you won't freeze in the face of anxiety. Instead, you'll take action.

Step Three is where you go on the offensive—taking back what the enemy has stolen by rewiring your mind to function on truth, not lies. It's not just about removing Satan's deception; it's about filling that space with God's Unshakeable Word.

Because once you've stripped the enemy's lies of their power and replaced them with truth, you have everything you need to walk in freedom.

This is where real transformation happens.

This is how you renew your mind and reshape your thinking—not just for a moment, but for a lifetime of victory over anxiety.

So the only question is, are you ready to walk in that freedom?

"So if the Son has set you free, you are free indeed!"

END NOTE

TIME TO REST

"The wise rest at least as hard as they work."
–Mokokoma Mokhonoana

~~~

You've made it to the finish line—bravo!

Now you have the game plan to crush anxiety, defeat overwhelm, and conquer the fears that freak you out. You've learned how to recognize the enemy's tactics, renounce his lies, and replace them with God's truth, stripping Satan of the power he once had over your life. You're no longer fighting empty-handed—you're armed, equipped, and ready to walk in freedom.

So what's the result?

REST.

Not just physical rest. Soul-deep, anxiety-free, heart-at-peace rest. The kind of rest where you're no longer fighting just to keep your head above water—you're walking confidently, no longer controlled by fear.

And that's exactly what Jesus promises us in Matthew 11:28:

"Come to me, all you who are weary and burdened, and I will give you rest."

That's the invitation. Not to work harder. Not to strive more. Not to prove yourself worthy. Just come to Him—with all your fears, all your struggles, and all your exhaustion—and let Him give you the rest your soul has been craving.

"For my yoke is easy and my burden is light" (Matthew 11:29).

Don't miss the word picture Christ gives us here. Imagine yourself plowing a field with an old wooden yoke strapped around your neck like the oxen in biblical times. You're sweating, your shoulders are raw, your legs are burning—it's brutal. Every step feels heavier than the last, and you're exhausted.

Then, you glance over and see Jesus plowing too. But He's not struggling. He's steady, strong, and completely at peace. He looks at you with kindness and says, *"Why don't you come over here and yoke up with Me? I think you'll find it much better."*

Without a second thought, you drop your yoke and step into His. And suddenly, everything changes. You're still plowing, still doing the work—but it's no longer crushing. The weight that once drained you now feels light. The burden that once exhausted you now feels manageable.

That's the beauty of yoking up with Jesus—He doesn't just give us rest; He *is* our rest. True, lasting, soul-deep rest.

Here's the truth:

Overcoming anxiety isn't about fighting harder. It's about surrendering better. It's not about mustering up more strength. It's about handing over the weight that was never yours to carry in the first place.

Every fear. Every expectation. Every overwhelming "what if."

When you stop clutching onto control and finally release it into Jesus' hands, something incredible happens—He carries it for you.

The steps we've given you—Recognize, Renounce, Replace—are powerful, but not because of the steps themselves. They are simply the process that connects you to the One who has the power.

And He's the One who gives you rest.

This is the freedom you've been searching for. The peace you've been craving.

So step into it. Live in it. Because you were never meant to live bound by anxiety.

You were made to be free.

A GIFT FOR YOU

As you close this book, we want to leave you with more than just encouragement—we want to equip you for the road ahead. That's why we've created a special gift just for you: a free digital download of a unique companion book we crafted for those who want to go deeper.

Over the course of a year, I (Jason) walked alongside a man battling anxiety, using the exact principles laid out in this book. We coached together through an online platform that captured our full conversation—every question, breakthrough, and real-time struggle. What unfolded was a powerful, raw, and deeply practical journey of transformation.

I've taken that coaching experience and put it into book format so you can see what it looks like to apply these truths day by day. It's not theory—it's lived-out, in-the-trenches work that shows how God meets us in our mess and walks us into peace.

This is our gift to you. It's honest. It's practical. And it's yours—completely free.

You'll find the download link at the end of this chapter. Our prayer is that it helps you take everything we've covered and lock it into your everyday life with courage and hope.

Visit JasonAndTori.com/AnxietyCoach

YOUR FIVE CORE NEEDS

*"Once our basic needs are satisfied,
our level of wealth has little to
no effect on how happy we are."*
–Unknown

I n Chapter 12, we discussed your #1 core human need—security. But we don't want to leave you hanging, wondering what the rest are.

So, as we wrap this book up, we want to give you a quick look at the core needs God wired into your DNA—the very things that drive you, shape you, and ultimately lead you to Him. I learned this from a good friend, Dr. Kathy Koch, in her amazing book, *FIVE TO THRIVE*.[51]

All people have five core human needs. They are:

- Security—*who can I trust?*

- Identity—*who am I?*

- Belonging—*who wants me?*

- Purpose—*why am I alive?*

- Competence—*what do I do well?*

As we discussed earlier, all the needs are built upon the first and primary need for security.

The very fabric of your life is built upon security. You learned it from the time you were an infant. When you cried, you learned to trust that your mom would meet your needs. This is why the mother-baby bond is so tight—it's forged on the foundation of trust.

If you grew up in a healthy family, you soon learned to trust your parents to provide for you and protect you. This gave you a sense of security, and from that place of safety ...

- You were able to discover who you were (identity).
- You knew you had a family who loved you no matter what (belonging).
- You understood that your life was significant and had meaning (purpose).
- You learned that you had gifts and talents that could help others (competence).

Can you see why the attack on the family is so detrimental today? Hollywood, big tech, secular media, and a host of streaming services push content that redefines this most basic foundation of humanity, and it has wreaked havoc on so many people.

These days, many people are growing up with no real sense of security, which has led to a host of other needs going unmet throughout their lives. Just turn on the news, and you'll see how destructive this anti-family worldview has become.

Our ultimate security can only be found in the one who created us— God. This is why there are so many verses in the Bible about trusting God. He wired us to connect with Him by trusting Him through His Son, Jesus Christ. When we do, everything we know and believe filters through that solid foundation.

Look at what Jesus said:

"... believe in the Light, so that you may become sons of the Light" (John 12:36).

Finding our security in Christ *changes who we are*. Placing our trust in Him changes our identity into one of God's kids.

This is life-changing. Placing our faith, hope, and trust in Christ sets the foundation for every other need in our lives to fall into place. Anxiety thrives when we feel unstable, uncertain, or unworthy—but when we allow God to meet our deepest needs, anxiety loosens.

Here's how it works:

- Security – *I trust God as my Father and Jesus as my Savior.*
- Identity – *I am a child of God; He's my Father.*
- Belonging – *God wants me because I'm His kid.*
- Purpose – *I want to bring my Father glory in all that I do.*
- Competence – *I can do all things through Christ who strengthens me.*

When your core needs are met in God, anxiety no longer has permission to control you. It doesn't matter what your past looked like, how your family treated you, or what the world says about you.

You are brand new. Transformed from the inside out. No longer striving, no longer searching—fully secure, fully loved, and finally at rest.

TOOLS TO HELP YOU KEEP WALKING IN FREEDOM

"Once our basic needs are satisfied, our level of wealth has little to no effect on how happy we are."
–Unknown

~~~

Breaking free from anxiety doesn't happen overnight. It's a daily walk, a mindset shift, and a spiritual battle all rolled into one. As you continue your journey beyond this book, here are some trusted resources that can equip you for the road ahead, and a cheat sheet when you need immediate help.

Use this list as a toolbox. Come back to it when you need strength, when you're struggling to stay steady, or when you just need a reminder that you're not alone, and that freedom really is possible.

Books

- **Anxious for Nothing** – *Max Lucado*
  A practical, encouraging look at Philippians 4 and how God's peace can guard our hearts and minds.

- **The Anxiety Cure** – *Dr. Archibald Hart*
  A foundational book from a Christian psychologist, exploring the physical, emotional, and spiritual sides of anxiety.

- **Get Out of Your Head** – *Jennie Allen*
  A powerful read on taking control of toxic thoughts and replacing them with God's truth.

- **Switch On Your Brain** – *Dr. Caroline Leaf*
  Neuroscience meets Scripture in this guide to renewing your mind and rewiring destructive patterns.

- **Winning the War in Your Mind** – *Craig Groeschel*
  My favorite book on the topic! It's a modern, faith-based guide to overcoming negative thought patterns and embracing truth.

- **Don't Give the Enemy a Seat at Your Table** – *Louie Giglio*
  A powerful reminder that fear and anxiety don't belong in your inner dialogue.

- **Running Scared** – *Edward T. Welch*
  A deeply biblical look at fear and anxiety from a counselor's perspective.

Apps & Tools

- **Abide App** – Christian meditation and sleep stories grounded in Scripture

- **Dwell App** – Listen to the Bible read aloud with calming music and voices

- **Pause App** – Developed to help you reset with guided pauses and prayer

Cheat Sheet

Back in Chapter Two, we talked about the sympathetic and parasympathetic nervous systems — basically your body's built-in gas pedal and brake. When anxiety hits, your foot slams the gas (sympathetic response). This cheat sheet will help you *tap the brakes* and shift back into a state of peace (parasympathetic).

WHEN YOU'RE STUCK IN SYMPATHETIC (FIGHT OR FLIGHT)

You might feel:

- Anxious, jittery, or wired
- Short of breath or tight chest
- Tense neck/shoulders
- Racing thoughts
- Irritable or reactive
- Digestive issues (bloating, upset stomach)
- Trouble sleeping

SWITCH TO PARASYMPATHETIC MODE WITH THESE TOOLS

1. BREATHING RESET

Technique: 4-7-8 Breath

- Inhale for 4 seconds
- Hold for 7 seconds
- Exhale slowly for 8 seconds
- Repeat 4 times

Why it works: Slows your heart rate and tells your brain "I'm safe."

2. PRAYER & MEDITATION (This is where Recognize, Renounce, Replace comes in)

Focus: Gratitude, trust, and God's presence

- Pray Psalm 46:10 – *"Be still and know that I am God."*
- Meditate on God's faithfulness — even 2–3 minutes calms the nervous system.

Why it works: Brings spiritual alignment and physiological peace.

3. COLD WATER SPLASH or SHOWER

- Splash cold water on your face or take a 30-second cold shower

Why it works: Activates the vagus nerve, which jumpstarts parasympathetic response.

4. WALK OUTSIDE (Preferably Barefoot or in Nature)

- 10–15 minutes of light walking, breathing deeply
- Get sunlight in your eyes (morning light is best)

Why it works: Combines movement, nature, and grounding — all parasympathetic boosters.

5. SLOW, LOW-INTENSITY MOVEMENT

- Stretching, yoga, or even gentle air squats/push-ups done slowly
- Add calming music

Why it works: Light movement without strain helps process cortisol without more stress.

6. PHYSICAL TOUCH (*Jason: I love this one!*)

- Hug your spouse, cuddle your kid, or pet your dog
- 20 seconds of safe touch = oxytocin release = instant calm

Why it works: It signals safety to your brain. Oxytocin = the "anti-cortisol" hormone.

7. LAUGH, SMILE, SING

- Watch a clean comedy clip
- Sing along to worship or upbeat music
- Smile on purpose (even if forced at first)

Why it works: All three activate the vagus nerve and pull you into parasympathetic mode.

8. CHEW GUM OR SLOWLY SIP WARM TEA

- Simple, but chewing or sipping signals "rest and digest"

Why it works: Mimics behaviors your brain associates with safety.

BONUS: STACK 2-3 OF THESE FOR FASTER RESULTS!

Example: Morning walk + prayer + sunlight
Or: Cold shower + breathwork + worship music

Now go and enjoy your freedom!

ENDNOTES

1   Dr. Tony Evans, *The Tony Evans Bible Commentary* (Hebrews 12:25-27)

2   Dr. John Gottman, *The Seven Principles That Make Marriage Work*

3   Craig D. Lounsbrough

4   Max Lucado, *Anxious For Nothing*

5   The Message Bible

6   Hart, Archibald D. *Adrenaline and Stress*. W Publishing Group, 1995 / The Anxiety Cure. Thomas Nelson, 2001.

7   National Library of Medicine. https://www.ncbi.nlm.nih.gov/books/NBK279390/

8   Waxenbaum, Joshua A., Vamsi Reddy, and Matthew A. Varacallo. *Anatomy, Autonomic Nervous System*. StatPearls Publishing. January, 2025.

9   LeWine, Howard E., MD. *Understanding The Stress Response*. Harvard Health Publishing. April, 2024

10 For more information, visit www.Health.com

11 Dictionary.com

12 Dictionary.com

13 Jon Gordon, *The One Truth*

14 Seward, Zachary M. "An average NFL game: more than 100 commercials and just 11 minutes of play." Published on QZ.com 11-24-2013.

15 https://www.bodyandsoul.com.au/nutrition/gut-health/5-foods-that-trigger-anxiety-according-to-a-nutritional-psychiatrist/news-story/9a7044a3b16a44423b391d9e5c2a1782

16 Dictonary.com

17 Oxford Dictionary

18 Skip Moen, in *Today's Word* - https://skipmoen.com/todays-word/

19 *Blondin: His Life and Performances*. Edited by G. Linnaeus Banks. London, New York: Routledge, Warne, and Routledge, 1862.

20 Oxford Dictionary / Merriam-Webster Dictionary

21 American social psychologist Roy Baumeister - https://www.youtube.com/watch?v=KfnUicHDNM8

22 Duhigg, Charles. *The Power of Habit: Why We Do What We Do in Life and Business*. Random House, 2012.

23 Dictionary.com

24 Logos Bible Word Study Guide

25   Merriam-Webster Dictionary

26   Jesse Johnson, "Why We Sing 'I Have Decided to Follow Jesus.'" *The Cripplegate.* May 29, 2013.

27   American Psychological Association. https://www.apa.org/monitor/2012/10/solitary

28   Dr. Cloud has noted that he has looked and looked for the source on the study on monkeys but has been unable to locate the original research.

29   Original quote attributed to Christine Lee

30   Kenyon, Kathleen M. *Digging Up Jericho: The Results of the Jericho Excavations,* 1952–1956. London: Praeger, 1957

31   Skip Moen, *Today's Word*

32   https://pmc.ncbi.nlm.nih.gov/articles/PMC3827523/

33   Andy Stanley, *Visioneering*

34   https://positivepsychology.com/neuroscience-of-gratitude/

35   Oswald Chambers, *My Utmost For His Highest*

36   Mayo Clinic. "Helping People, Changing Lives: 3 Health Benefits Of Volunteering." *Speaking Of Health* newsletter. August 1, 2023.

37   Dictionary.com

38   https://pmc.ncbi.nlm.nih.gov/articles/PMC9954474/

39   Dr. Daniel Amen, *You, Happier*

40   https://www.mdpi.com/2254-9625/14/3/40

41   Dr. Andrew Huberman, Huberman Lab Podcast

42   https://adaa.org/living-with-anxiety/managing-anxiety/exercise-stress-and-anxiety

43   https://pmc.ncbi.nlm.nih.gov/articles/PMC9254653/

44   Dr. Archibald Hart, *Adrenaline And Stress*

45   Unknown

46   Oswald Chambers, *My Utmost For His Highest*

47   Quote attridubted to John Green

48   Dr. Caroline Leaf, *Switch On Your Brain*

49   Dictionary.com

50   https://www.scientificamerican.com/article/caterpillar-butterfly-metamorphosis-explainer/

51   Learn more about Dr. Koch at www.CelebrateKids.com